At Our Age

How to Make 50 - 90 Your Dynamite Years

by

Dianne Peck

© 2004 by Dianne Peck. All rights reserved.

No part of this book may be reproduced, stored in a retrieval system, or transmitted by any means, electronic, mechanical, photocopying, recording, or otherwise, without written permission from the author.

First published by AuthorHouse 09/17/04

ISBN: 1-4184-6889-4 (e-book)
ISBN: 1-4184-3137-0 (Paperback)

This book is printed on acid free paper.

Acknowledgements

I greatly desire to acknowledge my wonderful Life Coach, Dawn, who brilliantly charted the course for me from the too-familiar shore of closet writer, safely across unknown waters to the exhilarating shore of published author. I also acknowledge International Coach Academy where I first received coaching for my terror at getting published.

Dedication

Because at our age friends are a great treasure, I dedicate this book to

Marguerite, a trusted confidante

Janet, who validates me as a creative

Mary, who assures me I am a leader

Dianna, who validates my spirituality

Sis, who holds my vision for me always

Leone, steadfast friend for more than forty years

Tony, who made a long road bend

Sheila, for whom mysticism is everyday fare

Contents

Chapter	Page
Chapter One You're How Old?...............................	1

You're the perfect age

Chapter Two Transitions	21

Making it through

Chapter Three The "S" Word (Stress).........................	45

Riding the crest of the wave

Chapter Four Let's Play Again, Sam...........................	67

The right age for fun

Chapter Five At the Ready..	87

Falling in love

Chapter Six Sex – At Our Age?	111

Better than ever

Chapter Seven Getting the Money You Want	137

Here's how

Chapter Eight Oh But You Can...................................	159

Create the life you want

Appendix A Taking Action...	181

Appendix B   The Power of Allowing 187

Appendix C   Life Coaching 195

Chapter One
You're How Old?

Growing old is no more than a bad habit
which a busy person has no time to form.
Andre Maurois

The absolute truth is this: You aren't past your "Best Before" date. Would you like to read that again? Here it is: You aren't past your "Best Before" date.

For instance, just this week the clock radio started my day with an interview with scientist Sir Joseph Rotblat who was in town as Keynote speaker for the Pugwash Movement, an anti-nuclear movement of which he is the Founder.

Dianne Peck

Nobel Peace Prize winner in 1995, he was promoting the movement's long term goal, which is the end of all war as an institution. And he was promoting its short-term goal, the end of the nuclear arms race, which he expects to see in his lifetime. The point is this: Sir Joseph Rotblat is 95 years old.

How do you feel about your age? Have you had one of those birthdays, you know, the one they call "the big one"? If you're 49 the big one is 50. If you're 59 the big one is 60. And when your 89 the big one is 90…etc. How did you feel about "the big One"? Some of the clues to how our society feels are phrases such as "the big one". Just why is turning 59 or 69 or 89 "big"?

When we call it the "big one" we imply a variety of foreboding notions. Some of these are: there's no going back now; the best is behind; it's all downhill from here; I've had my moment on center stage and it's backstage from here on; my dimmer switch is stuck in the on position, and so on.

Most of us have inhaled this fatalistic faux-thinking since early childhood. For example, at the age of six I had my tonsils removed. My dominant memory is waking up in the recovery room next to a woman who was not handling the experience as zestfully as I was. She assured me I was the lucky one because "when you have youth you have everything".

Don't believe it. You aren't past your best before date, not at 50, not at 60, not at 90, not ever. William Sadler has filled his book, *The Third Age: 6 Principles of Growth and Renewal After Forty,* with very convincing data to prove this theory.

Sadler spent twelve years studying and researching the topic of growth in men and women between the ages of forty and eighty. The point of his book is that we are in a longevity revolution. The human life span now reaches into our 90's and 100's.

The author's question is, what are we doing with all those extra years? Are they just more years in which to be old? Or are they a not-to-be-missed opportunity for vibrant, creative, exciting living?

If not, why not? Who told us there is a point beyond which we are past our prime? And an even more penetrating question is: Why do we believe them?

We can have a thriving second-half-of-life experience. We just need to change the way we think about "growing old". We just need to change our mind. We just need to orchestrate a simple mind-revolution. We just need a few replacement thoughts.

The "D" words

We need to trade in the D-words, which the author of *The Third Age* lists as decline, disease, dependency, depression, decrepitude, and the biggest D-word, death. They do not paint a pretty picture. They do not create one iota of life for the person thinking them, or for the person listening to the person who is thinking them when she/he starts speaking them.

At Our Age

In fact, if you use the current norm for the onset of middle age, which has gratuitously been upped from 35 to 40, and the current norm for our lengthening years, which is 90, then you are living 55% of your lifetime under the gathering clouds of the D-words.

One of the problems with this mindset is that its messages are so subtle. You don't notice them right away, then one day you realize your self-esteem is floundering, or you've lowered the bar for your personal performance expectations, or "I'm getting too old for that kind of thing" are words that begin to escape your lips on a regular basis.

You start identifying with jokes such as, "I'm at an age when a short pencil is better than a long memory", or my favorite, "you know you're old when you bend over to tie your shoe and look around to see what else you can do while you're down there".

The "R" words

The idea that we can stop accepting the conventional messages that our culture promotes about aging, that we can create an alternate approach to life after fifty, is good news. I'm excited about it. I'm believing it and I'm acting on it. I'm making it the focus of my energy because trading in the D-words for R-words feels good. Sadler's R-words are beautiful words like renewal, rebirth, reinvention, regeneration, and revitalization.

These concepts are not new to the cosmetic manufacturers. You can find bottles labeled Rejuvenation and other R-words at any cosmetic counter. But it's the renewal and revitalization of our thought processes that will allow us to live our lengthened days with joy.

So just how do we begin to change our mind?

The process is called re-framing and it means getting a new perspective on an old thought.

At Our Age

The first re-framing I did for myself was to toss away the term "middle age" and replace it with the term "Third Age". An updated classification of our human growth stages goes like this:

- the First Age of our lives is the learning stage, from birth to approximately age twenty;
- the Second Age is the onset of productivity when we form careers, establish families, etc and lasts from age twenty to age forty, approximately;
- the Third Age is called the growth stage, and spans the years from forty to eighty (that's right, from forty to eighty, approximately);
- the Fourth Age is the successful aging process from eighty to…approximately.

At our age we are in the enviable position of having life launch us into a forty-year period of new growth. We don't have to launch ourselves. Life leads the way, then looks back at us and beckons. Come over here, life says. Walk this way, life says. Go there, life says.

All we have to do is put one foot in front of the other, just once. All we have to do is take the first step, then that step multiplies itself, and autopilot clicks on. The D words are no longer in the forefront of our thinking. The R words become our reality and we are launched into our new perspective, and therefore into our new life.

Create the life you want

Because perspective is everything, I would like to share some of the insights about it which are revolutionizing my life.

How we view a situation determines the results we get. That is the same as saying that we can create our own outcome. Yes, that is what I am saying. We can create the life we want.

This theory hunted me down. It seemed that every author I read was promoting it and I finally began to get it. It had become one of those "come over here" leads from life.

This is what I have come over to:

Thoughts are electro-magnetic energy. We have the backing of the Quantum Physicists, lead by Albert Einstein, on that, so I felt fairly secure in pursuing more.

Our thoughts are magnets and like magnets, they follow the same natural law as the rest of the electric-magnetic energy in the Universe. They draw like unto like. Simply put, positive and life-giving thoughts create positive and life-giving reality.

Quantum Physics belongs to this century but awareness of the power of thought began a couple of millennia ago.

The Buddha said, "We are what we think. All that we are arises with our thoughts. With our thoughts we make our world".

Plato said, "Take charge of your thoughts. You can do what you will with them".

In 1921 Genevieve Behrend wrote, in *Your Invisible Power*, "Try to remember that the picture you think, feel, and see is reflected into the Universal Mind, and by natural law of reciprocal action must return to you in either spiritual or physical form".

In 1937 Napoleon Hill wrote, in *Think and Grow Rich*, "Truly thoughts are things, and powerful things at that when they are mixed with definiteness of purpose, persistence, and a burning desire for their translation into riches or other material objects".

Too good to be true, I said, but it isn't. Our perspective, that is, our thoughts and our feelings about a particular circumstance, situation, problem, challenge, event, relationship, development etc. is either a positive one or a negative one. And it will produce like results. Yes, if we focus on what we want, it will come to us.

Become aware of your current perspective. If it is all about what you don't want or don't have, re-frame it into a picture of what you want.

Focus on the outcome you want. Feel it. Act as if you already have it. Then sit back and let life show you how to receive it. Let life guide you in the steps you need to take to get it.

New perspectives

What are some perspectives we need to develop for our Third Age, our growth age? What are some of the new mindsets that will take us where we want to go?

-1- the "I'm not what I used to be" replacement.

No, you're not what you used to be. For one thing, you literally do not have the body you had because almost every cell has been replaced. That is a process that takes place several times during your lifespan. And you do not have the mind or emotions you had because life has mde you more experienced, wiser, softer, more malleable, smarter, and more intuitive.

The circumstances of your life are changing, perhaps relentlessly. For example, some of the roles you have played have changed. Maybe your children are raised, you've retired from your career, or you've endured the passing of your parents or other loved ones. The old frame said, "I don't recognize my life anymore." The new frame says, "I have a new-found freedom."

Now you are free to be responsible for you. Now you are the focus of your role as provider and parent and caregiver. Now you can gather in all that lived experience and shower it on you.

At Our Age

What new opportunities do you want to explore? What new role do you want to play? What new lifestyle do you want to live? What loving work awaits you? Who needs what you have to give? What new doors await your knock?

Leading scholar Joseph Campbell repeatedly said, "Follow your bliss".

He defined bliss as "that deep sense of being at the very center…and doing what the push is out of your own existence. You follow that and doors will open where there were no doors…where you never thought there were going to be doors, and where there wouldn't be a door for anybody else…" (from a Joseph Campbell television series).

When you are in the Third Age, growth means not being what you used to be because it means becoming a new creation. The word "retirement" is from the French "re", which means from, and "tirer" which means to pull or draw.

We need to retire the word "retirement". Our general understanding is just that, retirement is a withdrawing from, a pulling back from. No, no, no. We are not pulling back from, we are pivoting, gently adjusting our compass to a new direction.

It isn't a retirement program; it is a re-entry program. We are re-entering our lives, this time with our own fulfillment, our completion, and ourselves as our main responsibility. "For the first time in the human experience, we have the chance to shape our new work to suit the way we want to live…we would be mad to miss the chance". Charles B. Handy

No, you aren't what you used to be because you no longer want to be. What you are now is a pioneer and an explorer on the frontier of fabulous growth. The purpose of your younger years was to take you to now, to these growth years, "the last of things for which the first was made", as Robert Browning put it.

-2- Write your own script

Another characteristic of your third Age, which you are most likely very aware of already, is your need to question the script you live by. If you have not begun critiquing this script yet, you will find yourself doing so. You will find yourself questioning the guidelines that have been written inside your mind and that have dictated the way you have lived your life.

What you are asking yourself now is, who wrote them? Did I or did others? Are they good for me? Do they still fit me? Do they still hold true for the person I am becoming? Do I keep them or do I re-write them?

The following incident is trivial in its circumstances but illustrates the point.

When I was about six I had devoured an apple down to the core and wanted to know what parts of the core were edible. "Is it alright to eat the fuzzy end?" I foolishly asked my older brother. "Sure", he said, "that's the best part".

Not detecting the teasing in his voice, I dutifully consumed the blossom end of the apple, for years. Then one day, to my credit, I questioned the advice and rejected it in favor of my common sense.

The Third Age brings us to our common sense.

It is a major breakthrough in our personal growth when we reflect on all the standards, codes, restrictions, and behaviors with which we have been programmed by society, by our family of origin, and by the major institutions in our educational and religious background. We sort through them. We discard some and we keep others, and some we revamp and make our own.

A friend reports that as she comes into this awakening, as she wakes up to herself, she has a wild desire to walk out of her current life completely and create a brand new free and flowing one. I say, go for it.

In fact, examples of folks who have leaped into new lives (with fewer or greater degrees of wild abandon) may be all around you.

A tourist attraction in the town next to mine is the Glace Bay Miner's Museum. It contains an exhaustive depiction of the three hundred million-year history of coal formation in the earth, and the two hundred and eighty-one year history of local mining. (The first commercial coal mining operation began locally in Port Morien, NS. in 1720, with the double significance of being the first systematic way of mining coal on the North American continent).

The museum also contains a real coalmine through which a mine guide does just that, guides, informs and leads you. No cosmetics have been applied to the underground experience. You are escorted through the stark, cruel, and primitive conditions in which the early miners labored.

Our mine guide's name was Hinson Calabrese, a

former miner. Nimble and smart and witty, he re-entered life as a mine guide 17 years ago. Only a cane, necessitated by an old mining injury, gave any hint of his 83 years.

Welcome yourself to Third Age, because it is the time when we have new tools for making choices. It is the time when we are free to take risks, surge forward, explore new horizons, and advance our personal fulfillment.

The goal of this book is to make you an expert in the use of one tool in particular and that tool is the power of your own thoughts.

The following chapters will explore the ways in which our thought life can bring dynamic living to the major areas of our lives, including life transitions, stress, fun, falling in love, sex, and money.

RESOURCES

The Third Age: 6 Principles for Growth and Renewal After Forty. William A. Sadler. Perseus Publishing, Cambridge, Mass. 2000.

Let Your Life Speak. Parker J. Palmer. Jossey-Bass, San Francisco, Cal. 2000.

Seven Spiritual Laws of Success: A Practical Guide to the Fulfillment of Your Dreams. Deepak Chopra, Publishers Group. 1996

Manifest Your Destiny. Wayne Dyer. Harper Collins, New York. 1999.

Chapter Two
Transitions

The Universe oozes with power, waiting for anyone who wishes to embrace it.
Brian Swimme

Change your mind and you change your world.

On the one hand it seemed several years in coming, on the other, suddenly there it was. I was not only living alone, but also was solely responsible, for the first time in my life, for my own finances, for procuring an income.

Until now, my economic contribution to the household had been in the form of services. You know, cook, nurse, chauffeur, babysitter, housecleaner, secretary, instructor, keeper of traditions, nest builder, etc. Bringing home a paycheck had not been part of my job description.

But that's the thing about life, it changes. Whether we want it to or not, whether we're paying attention or not, it changes. Circumstances jump up and take over our lives and life is suddenly challenging us with a major transition.

Life transitions

Transitions can have different faces.

They can come in the form of the loss of a job, or the beginning of a new one; forced or chosen retirement from a lifelong career; the end of a relationship or the beginning of one; the death of a loved one; the need to move to a new geographical location; the onset of an illness or disability that is changing life as we knew it. They can come because people disappoint us or dreams don't materialize.

Transitions can make us feel as if everything that gave life meaning, our health, our money, our job, our relationships, and even our potential, is rapidly getting downsized.

It's about then that our human reactions take over.

They can run the gamut from fear, denial, anger, resentment and resistance, to procrastination and paralysis. It is natural to fear and dread the day when "something happens" to change the familiarity, routine, and sense of safety that go with being able to maintain our life's status quo. That is because we equate the word "transitions" with another frightening word, "endings".

Yes, transitions are endings. And endings connote a mindset of finality, loss, grief, gone-forever, never-again. A fearing, confused, what-to-do-now, this really hurts, I'm scared, I don't want to go on, mindset. Even a - this shouldn't have happened, I never wanted this to happen, I'm cut to the quick, I'm very, very angry, mindset. That is when change feels like it's going to kill us and life becomes very raw.

But transitions are also another experience called beginnings. And beginnings connote a newness, anticipation, growth, first-time excitement, clear-crisp-air mindset. A greening, surging forward, pioneering, get-it-right-this time, better-than-ever, second-time-lucky, age-doesn't-mean-a-thing, clean-slate mindset.

Transitions are a dual-sided phenomenon. The challenge comes in not taking up residence in Side A, endings. The challenge is to taste those endings as fully as possible, and then to walk away into the spectacular new day that is waiting, that is tailor made for you and your future.

Let's take a closer look at that.

To taste the full impact of the ending that has come, bidden or unbidden, into your life, means to feel exactly what you are feeling. Here are some ways to do that.

#1: <u>The OK List</u>: (getting through survival mode)

Get pen and paper and at the top write "My OK List".

Now list each feeling, thought and belief you have about the transition that you face. Be completely honest here. Don't feel you have to cover up the biggies such as hate, revenge, resentment, paralyzing fear, depression, guilt, doubt, etc. Take time with this; do it in a few sittings if you need to. Your goal is to simply name the feelings, reactions, and thoughts you are experiencing.

You now have an OK List. This is called an OK List because now you are going to give everything on your list permission to be there. Yes, permission.

The thing is this. Our human response to the presence of what has been called our shadow side is to judge it, and to judge it harshly. If we put a "you shouldn't feel or think that way" judgment on our thoughts and feelings, we add a layer of self-bashing to our already throbbing mind and heart.

When we censor ourselves in this way, what we are actually doing is invalidating ourselves. We are invalidating our humanness. Your reactions to the endings in your life are neither right nor wrong. They are true to the human nature that you come with.

Respect your list

So what you do is this. The opposite of invalidation is respect, so now you are going to take each item on your OK List and respect it. One by one, respect each frightening thought, emotion, and belief. Gently sit with the fear (anger, depression, confusion etc.) and say, "Fear (anger etc.) it is OK that you are here."

Go all the way

Go a step further. Say, "Fear (anger etc), I welcome you."

Now go all the way. Put your arms around it. Gather it in to you. Thank it for being with you and ask it to release its gift to you. This process may sound bizarre if you are encountering it for the first time. Thank my problem for being in my life? No way!

Here is what some best-selling authors say about this process.

Author Deepak Chopra says, "…the shadow energies never had a chance to show you their hidden message…as soon as you do that they will deliver their message and then go" (from *The Deeper Wound*).

Author Clarissa Estes says that when we take in our troublesome emotion with compassion we "render it for our own constructive use"(from *Women Who Run With The Wolves*).

In Buddhist teaching this OK-ing process is the art of loving-kindness practiced on yourself. Buddhist author Pema Chodron, in her book *The Places That Scare You*, uses the analogy of the mother bird protecting and feeding her "naked, squeaking, homely babies".

We find we are both the chicks, homely and demanding in our hurt and pain, and the mother with her unconditional acceptance. We, too, can respond to our not-so-lovely inner offspring with unconditional loving kindness.

Be gentle

This is a gentle technique.

It is not about struggling to escape from the rowdy feelings. It is about sitting with them in love and compassion, befriending them, and receiving their gift. And what is their gift? When you give them what they are looking for, a rightful place with you, they calm down. Like chicks, they grow up. They become tools and helpers and promoters.

And their gift is that all of their energies are transformed for you to use in whatever way you need. Your fatigue goes and you feel supported on every side with energies you hardly recognize.

My current challenge is to adjust to living alone.

Coming home to an empty apartment can sting. I step in and it hits, not unlike a sharp slap in the face. At other times the solitude, day and night, (I work from home which can fuel a sense of isolation) feels like a tidal wave that is threatening to wash me away.

There is also the challenge of creating a viable income, which, every now and then, brings with it an old friend of mine, insomnia.

Yes, endings can hurt and they can alter and complicate our life. A great deal of our energy will go into surviving them.

But the good news is that we do not have to stay in survival mode. We absolutely must not stay in survival mode. We must move through survival mode and into Side B of the transition experience. And what is Side B? Side B is thriving mode.

Your right to thrive

To thrive means to prosper outstandingly; to grow vigorously; to advance successfully. (Encyclopedia Britannica).

What do you believe about your right to thrive?

Check closely. You may actually believe that you don't deserve to thrive. You may believe that getting by is more in line with what you deserve.

Consider this. Thriving is our inheritance. Prospering outstandingly is our natural state. Scientists tell us that abundance is the way of the Universe. And we need only to look up at the galaxies, out over oceans, or ahead over mountains and forests and prairies to see the proof.

I love the line from the Talmud that says, "Every blade of grass has its angel that bends over it and whispers, 'Grow. Grow'."

You and I have an angel bending over us and whispering, "Prosper, flourish, abound, advance, progress."

We do not have an angel whispering, "Barely survive". But we might have a limiting belief telling us that, one that has been hanging around since early childhood. Not to worry.

This is the thing about limiting beliefs: they can't survive once they are uncovered. They resist discovery, because discovery ends their reign, zaps them like a laser beam, so check your beliefs about your right to thrive. You could be the only thing holding you back

#2: <u>Success LifeLine</u>: (getting into survival mode)

Drawing my personal Success LifeLine was a suggestion from my Life Coach. A Life Coach is someone who helps you map out where you are trying to go, in my case, through an ending and into a beginning, and then walks with you until you get there, doing for you whatever it takes to keep you moving ahead and reaching the finish line.

You can find more information on professional Life Coaching at the end of this chapter, and in Appendix C at the end of this book.

A **Success LifeLine** works this way.

Draw a line across a page and mark in any successes you can remember, from earliest childhood until the present.

You can choose overall successes from you life, or

the successes from your past experiences that pertain to the issue at hand, in this case, life transitions.

My first marker was age nine. That was the year my family moved out of the city and into the wilderness (a child's perception). I remember sitting on the unfamiliar front steps, looking across the harbor at the city shoreline and crying for hours. I kept that up for about two weeks.

But my broken heart must have healed because the dominant memory now is of the glorious hours on the neighboring farm that were spent bringing the cows home, gathering eggs, holding fuzz-ball chicks, pulling carrots and radishes for snacks, and playing in the off-limits hayloft. The pain of the ending has yielded to the treasures of the new beginning.

This memory affirmed my innate courage, temporarily forgotten.

It also reminded me where my love for rural living, for the silence in nature, and for the natural cycle of life, which seem to have embedded themselves in my DNA, began.

The point of making a success line is to remind ourselves that we have indeed already successfully transitioned at other junctures in our lives and therefore we can do so again.

Other markers on my Success LifeLine were the high school years, teacher training, marriage, motherhood, empty nest, the death of my parents and brother, the changes that a partner's serious illness brings to a primary relationship, etc. Most of these are transition successes now.

The exercise of making a Success LifeLine can reduce your vat of helplessness to, let's say, bucket size, and give you a jumping off point for moving forward in the transition process.

#3: **Get Connected**: (staying in thriving mode)

Whatever the particular circumstances of your transition, it will help you to:

-a- Connect with other people.

I found the weekends overwhelming and only getting worse. Waiting for something to come up wasn't working.

Now I make sure I have at least one thing scheduled between Friday night and Monday morning. I visit. I force myself to take in a show, even if I go alone. I get myself invited to dinner with extended family. I cook dinner and take it to shut-in friends and eat it with them.

A side effect of my changed circumstances is a new identity. My new availability is giving me a new role in the lives of friends and family.

In the beginning of a transition you aren't sure who you are, but gradually two things happen.

-1- You recover who you were, and at the same time

-2- You become someone new.

For example, the upside of being responsible for no one but myself (translation: living alone) is that I have much greater freedom if I want to leave town, do a favor for someone, change a plan, or make or unmake a decision, and much more flexibility for living my life.

-b- Connect on-line.

If a computer terrifies you, I've been there. But with my adult children spread over three countries (and two continents), I had a reason for plunging ahead.

And how about this thought, "If you are alive, you are fearful. It is nothing new". (Clarissa Estes). Who told you that you couldn't learn to use a computer? Are you taking their word for it?

You need to learn only the most basic steps:

- how to turn on the machine (push a button),
- how to move the mouse (a few tries and you've got it…an eight year old taught me),
- how to connect to the Internet (a few more clicks),
- and how to send and get email (again, just a matter of a few clicks).

I am not exaggerating. You can do this.

Libraries do a fabulous job of getting you launched.

The Bill and Melinda Gates Library Foundation has provided your library with a computer lab and free instruction, and with computers for public use if you aren't ready to own your own.

I began my computer journey a few years ago at age fifty-seven with an Introductory course. Thought I'd feel conspicuously out of place in the group until the first class, when a particularly dynamite couple joined us. At age 84, he was the older of the two by a year.

Take yourself into a wonderful world where you can:

-1- connect with on-line communities of like-minded people,
-2- find endless information – even a zip code/postal code you need, or maybe the best long-distance telephone plan
-3- shop till you drop and never leave your chair
-4- send and receive email…friends, family, business colleagues… anywhere, anytime
-5- read or purchase books
-6- pay your bills
-7- book plane tickets and hotels at the lowest rates
-8- chat/date.

The list goes on. If you haven't taken the leap into

the Internet world, push past that fear and give it a try. It can substantially advance your transition experience.

Well-known author Louise Hay handled her initial dread of the computer this way. She reframed her perspective on it.

Now that it had become a necessary tool for her livelihood, she changed her belief that this piece of too-modern technology was the troll waiting under the bridge to devour her. She listed all the things that were right about what it was bringing into her life. Then she gave it a beautiful name. Her resistance came tumbling down and her business gained a new level of excitement.

#4: <u>Self-Care</u>: (thriving par excellence)

Self-care may be the most important element in your creating a successful transition.

Self-care means you deliberately put your physical, mental, emotional and spiritual health first.

This may not be something in which you are well practiced. Your ears may hear self-care, but your brain hears self-ish.

Ditch that conditioning immediately. Our absolute first responsibility is our own well being. This is a very old concept. The part of "love your neighbor as you love yourself" that hasn't gotten any press is "as you love yourself". It's time for you to give it some.

More than at any other time, the time of a transition is the right time to love yourself. Stop many times a day and ask what you can do in that moment to love yourself.

Do you need to:

-a- drop your tense shoulders

-b- let go of the sense of urgency that's giving you the headache

-c- step outside into fresh air or sunshine

-d- disable the phone,

-e- eat some good food

-f- drink water

-g- lie down,

-h- buy yourself something

-i- call a loved one

-j- go on a date with just you

-k- go away for a few days

-l- simplify your lifestyle

-m- have unadulterated fun for an hour

-n- bide your time

-o- sign up for a class you love

-p- join a cause

-q- say no

-r- meditate

-s- go for a walk

When you become serious about loving yourself, you will find every minute teeming with how-to's.

In *The Artist's Way*, author Julia Cameron tells us that through self-nurturance we nurture our connection to our inner Spirit, to Universe, to whomever the in-dwelling Greater Power is for each of us. And that connection is key. It is by knowing we are held together from the inside out that we will maneuver the rapids of our transition.

Care for yourself first. Nurture yourself. Love yourself. Then you will have a reservoir of love and care and nurturance for others.

At this moment what is your transition status? You might be on the edge of a transition you know you need to make, but you feel paralyzed to take the first step. You may be already in the center of a transition whirlwind you didn't want but couldn't prevent.

Trust the power you have inside. Trust the power of your mind. Get clear on exactly where you want to be in this transition process, focus on that briefly and frequently, let go of a time frame for the outcome, and get ready to receive your new life.

RESOURCES

The Artist's Way. Julia Cameron. Tarcher Putnam, New York. 1992.

The Deeper Wound. Deepak Chopra. Harmony Books, New York. 2001.

The Places That Scare You. Pema Chodron. Shambala, Boston and London. 2001.

Women Who Run With the Wolves. Clarissa Pinkola Estes. Ballantine Books, New York.!992/95.

Professional Life Coaching:

Life coaching is a new profession that is rapidly gaining momentum. A Life Coach plays a similar role to that of a music coach or an athletic coach, only the area targeted for success is any aspect of your life in which you want support, structure, guidance and help in reaching your goals.

To read more about Life Coaching read Appendix C, page 195.

To find out if having a Life Coach will help you with your life transition, go to my website at:

www.diannepeck.com

For contact information for other Life Coaches, type Life Coach into any Internet Search Engine.

Chapter Three
The "S" Word (Stress)

Nothing can bring you peace but yourself.
Ralph Waldo Emerson

Fifty years ago only bridges were stressed. If a bridge was showing signs of stress, it meant that it was exceeding its weight-bearing capacity and the engineers were hastily called in.

Today people are stressed. Just like a bridge, we can all too easily exceed our own weight-bearing capacity. We feel as if the big bad stress fiend is devouring us, and it is.

Stress is wear and tear on the body from the inside out.

A list of stress-produced illnesses is lengthy and the list of symptoms is lengthier.

The warning signs are familiar to all of us: headache, hair loss, appetite loss or gain, tight muscles, increased heart rate, panic attacks, skin rashes, grinding teeth, indigestion, insomnia, increased smoking or drinking, depression, withdrawal, and more. We feel as if we are in a downward spiral that can't be reversed.

But the truth is, we can spiral upward again. Stress can be controlled, and even turned into an advantage.

We forget that some stress is needed in everything we do.

Gravity is the stress that keeps the galaxies in their place. In our daily life, applied stress means we can open a jar of peanut butter or lift weights. Emotional stress can mean we are motivated to act. The dilemma occurs only when stress exceeds the level that is useful and productive.

The burning question then becomes, what to do about too much stress?

Ways to control stress

There are several familiar recommendations to control the stress level of daily living.

Physical exercise is at the top of the list. That is because the adrenaline that stress produces in our bodies has to be burned off before it starts causing damage "from the inside out".

Then there is
- getting enough sleep
- eating healthful foods
- simplifying your lifestyle

- controlling your thoughts in order to let go of worry
- doing more of what you love
- getting organized
- managing your money
- meditation

Each of these suggestions is important and has a powerful effect on reducing our stress levels.

I am going to address two of them in more detail.

-1- Controlling your thoughts

A few years ago I got serious about money management and took a course in it. The first requirement of the course was that we observe. Everyday we observed what we were spending money on and kept a record. The process was enlightening. "I'm spending that much on _____? I had no idea!"

At Our Age

Taking inventory is also the place to start with thought management.

Begin to observe your thoughts. That's all, just notice them. Don't judge them or get upset about them, just notice them. You'll probably be enlightened. You'll probably say, "I'm spending that much energy on _____!" (Ex. Self-bashing, worrying, blaming, expecting the worst, etc).

We all have mind traps that are set and ready to spring.

For example, the thought "I can't do anything right", just because you couldn't do that one thing right.

Or "I know the boss has it in for me" because you didn't get the promotion.

Or, "Yes, I did that well, but I usually don't" when you are paid a compliment. And so we go.

My wake up call came not that long ago while I was reading a small book by Dr. Joe Vitale called *Spiritual Mar-*

keting.

In it the author reminds us about a very old theory that I have already mentioned a little earlier in this book, and it goes like this.

You can create the life you want. You can create what you want to have. You can change all those circumstances that you worry about, in fact, it is relatively easy to do. All you have to do is change your mind. Basically, that's it. And we're already quite adept at changing our mind; we do it all the time.

If you have already begun to note what kind of thoughts are in your mind, you are in the perfect position to get started on your mind-makeover.

Some of the thoughts I observed on myself go like this: "I am responsible for the happiness of my loved ones." "I need to perform perfectly." "I feel guilty because my son's marriage broke up…"etc.

The question you are asking yourself right now may be, "So what's the problem? Why do these thoughts need to be changed? They're just run of the mill human thoughts, aren't they?"

These thoughts need to be changed because, as we have already recalled, thoughts are energy, electro-magnetic energy. The power of thought is only beginning to strike home for us. The more positive the thought the more positive the results it produces.

We become what we think.

Focus on what you want

How do we harness this creative energy that fills every cell in our bodies? All that is required is that we think the right thoughts, that we focus on the outcome we want instead of the unwanted outcome we have or on the one we dreadfully anticipate, the "what if" one.

Ask yourself what you are focused on.

Someone said worry is focusing on what you don't want. When you catch yourself in panic mode, swing your mind over to the thought of what you want instead of the thought that is tearing you up.

Write it down and put it where you will bump into it frequently.

If we are focused on the best possible outcome, on the desire of our hearts, we clear a path for our desire to come to us. We draw it to us. And our stress level stays in a healthy and safe range.

I know a story about a woman who shed cigarette smoking by just this process.

She began by focusing on herself as a non-smoker instead of as a smoker. Anytime she didn't have a cigarette in her hand, she regarded herself as a non-smoker. And for that moment she was.

Gently, without great stress or tension, or the amping up of great amounts of will-power, her non-smoker periods increased. And she gradually and successfully became what she continuously focused on.

Feel as if

There is something else you can do to put the fullest amount of power behind your thoughts and that is, support them with your feelings.

Feel as if you already have what you need.

What will it feel like to be debt free? What will it feel like to have financial security for the rest of your life? What will it feel like to have a fulfilling relationship?

Feel those feelings now. Several times a day think of what you desire to create, such as financial security, feel the feelings that go with it, and hold them for half a minute or so. That's all there is to it. Oh yes, when you write out your goal, write it in the present, not the future. Write, "I have total financial security for the rest of my life", not "I am going to have total financial security for the rest of my life".

Letting go

There is one last step to facilitate this process.

It is the practice of letting go.

It is not a practice we hear much about in everyday circles, but it is the way to harness the power of your mind.

You have clearly defined what it is you want to create in your life. You feel it as if it is already here and you have written it as if it is already here.
Now do something that is called, "detaching from the outcome". Let go of deciding how your desire will

come to you, who will make it happen, and when it needs to happen.

For example, someone owes you $500. Your desire is that you get your money back.

Open yourself to every possibility. Your $500 will come to you, but not necessarily from the source you have determined. It's the "cast your bread upon the waters" phenomenon in operation. You are open and ready to receive from whichever wave brings it back to you.

Do not stop desiring, but let go of anxiety and worry. Relax into trust.

Go about your life as if you know a great secret, because you do. You know, before the evidence is there for all to see, that you already have the desire of your heart.

-2- Meditation

Meditation is a wide-ranging concept.

It is the experience of pondering and reflecting. And at the same time, as the pundit says, "Meditation. It's not what you think."

There are several different meditation techniques, but only one goal.

The goal of meditation is always to connect us to our Center, to the quiet Center in each of us, which is always there. Sometimes our Center is like the eye of the storm, surrounded by wild winds and turbulence. Meditation is the boat that carries us over the choppy waters, through the hurricane, and into the stillness.

We have a still Center and it is in that place that all the solutions to all our problems lie.

Oriah Mountain Dreamer, in her newest book, *The Call*, reminds us that there is nowhere we have to go to find what we need because it is right there at our Center. "Open the fist clenched in wanting and see what you already hold in your hand", she writes.

At times we may need someone to remind us to get into the boat, or to point the boat in the right direction for us, which is inward, where the answers are.

But at our Center is all our natural resourcefulness; eons of untapped potential is there. For every problem you have, your deep Center has an answer. The world's major corporations know that meditation is a highly effective tool for accessing that deep Center and those answers. That is why, on a regular basis, they sponsor "Retreat" weekends, management and staff included.

There are many ways to travel from outside ourselves where stress is battering us to inside ourselves where the stillness is.

Anything you do which gets you there is meditation.

Whatever you do to give yourself even a few moments of respite, of feeling good, of connecting to your true Self, is a meditation practice.

For one woman it is hanging out the clothes. Yes, and easy to see why.

"There I am", she says, "in the sunlight and fresh air, often in a soft breeze, doing clean work my hands love the feel of…". And her unconscious response is to immediately connect to her inner retreat space.

For a man I know, it is going fishing in the quiet and stillness of his secret fishing retreat.

Give yourself a Retreat hour or afternoon or evening or even a whole day.

Your meditation technique can be listening to music, having the house to yourself, puttering with a hobby, walking, writing in your journal, bringing something from nature indoors (one long winter I was feeling desperate for an indoor nature connection so I kept a snowball in the freezer), making love to yourself, having a massage, having a beautiful dinner for one, soaking in a bath, sitting in nature, practicing a formal meditation technique, and on.

Just when am I supposed to find time for this, you ask?

Well, there's the thing. What we're talking about here is controlling stress. It is vital to your health that you find the time so schedule yourself in. Pencil yourself into your day planner at least once a week for whatever time frame you can.

And bring no one with you. Connecting to your inner Self is a job for one.

Breathing

A simple but very effective way to loosen the tension and begin the shift to relaxation is by breathing.

Do this: (You can do it anywhere, and it takes only a few minutes).

-1- Drop your shoulders and tell your body to relax into whatever is supporting it, the chair, the bed, the floor, the earth.
-2- Breathe in from your abdomen for a count of four (you should be able to see your abdomen rise).
-3- Hold the breath for a count of four.
-4- Exhale for a count of eight.

Repeat this a few times.

Notice how tension leaves your body and how your mind can focus again. A breathing exercise is effective as a tool to slow you down in the middle of too-busy, or to escort you into meditation mode.

Morning Pages

I want to tell you about my current meditation practice. It is my greatest find. It is called the practice of morning pages.

It is simply a matter of going aside every day and writing three pages. Yes, three is the magic number, according to the creator of this technique, Julia Cameron in her book, *The Artist's Way*.

What do I write about?

Nothing and everything. That is the point. It is a kind of stream of consciousness writing. You just pick up the pen and start.

It might look like this, "Gotta get the groceries before I go to pick up John. Don't know how I'm going to fit everything in today. Feeling overwhelmed and haven't even started yet. So. What about this feeling of being overwhelmed. Not a stranger these days….feel it most in the evening…"

You just write. Anything. After a page or so there you are sailing along, and after a half hour or so you have filled three pages.

That's the first thing you notice.

What you also begin to notice is that you no longer feel overwhelmed. You feel put together and ready. You feel stilled and refreshed. Very gently your writing has taken you into your Center where your needs, even needs you weren't aware you had, were resolved without effort.

The only effort you exert is to write. Just pick up a pen and start writing, write anything that comes into your mind.

At Our Age

What happens is this. Your pages take you into your deep soul, who puts her arms around you and holds you more tenderly than you have ever been held. Who floods your "overwhelm" with extreme love.

I frequently have to pause, pen suspended, while I let a profound insight register or a long-sought answer assure me it is here.

Morning pages do not rake you over the coals of blame, do not drop you into the throbbing places or into the unbearable memories. They do not access your hurts and stand you naked in front of them to re-live them.

Morning pages access your Soul, your deep center where invisible arms hold you and unconditional love floods you.

The Universe always chooses the easy way. You can believe this. You can trust in this promise.

If meditation has not been part of your day, give this method a try.

We meditate because "guidance comes in advance of need". Do not be unsettled by the word "meditation". It is simply a tool to take you to where all the guidance you desire for your life is waiting for you, even before you need it.

RESOURCES

The Artisit's Way. Julia Cameron; Tarcher Putman, New York, NY. 1992.

Writing Down the Bones. Natalie Goldberg; Shambala, Boston, Mass. 1986.

The Power of Your Unconscious Mind. Joseph Murphy; Prentice Hall original edition. 1963.Bantam revised edition. 2001. USA and Canada.

The Power of Now. Eckhart Tolle; Namaste Publishing, Vancouver, BC. 1997.

The Call. Oriah Mountain Dreamer: Harper Collins, Toronto, Ont. 2003.

Don't Just Do Something, Sit There. Sylvia Boorstein; HarperCollins Canada. 1996.

www.meditationcenter.com

Chapter Four
Let's Play Again, Sam

At the height of Laughter, the universe is flung into a kaleidoscope of new possibilities.

Jean Houston

As I approached the corner store the other day I was jolted out of serious adult preoccupation by a young rollerblader making a hasty exit.

It wasn't the fact that he was on skates that drew me into the moment, as much as the ice-cream cone he was devouring. Just how long was it since I had lost myself in the pure delight of a double-decker chocolate ice cream cone?

I couldn't answer my own question because I couldn't remember when…I was talking years, here.

And let's not underestimate the importance that ice cream plays in our lives. Take that television commercial, for example, the one set in a psychiatrist's office and featuring the fellow who grew up in a family that couldn't afford ice cream. According to the commercial, here he is still miserable at age forty-nine, because he hasn't been able to give himself permission, even though he can well afford it, to buy himself an ice-cream cone.

So. No more self-imposed misery for me, no more running the risk of ending up on the psychiatrist's couch.

I promptly took remedial action and I don't know what felt better, the hedonistic pleasure of the ice cream or the almost forgotten feeling of "this is fun!"

It won't serve any purpose to lament our adult practice of abandoning the fun that was so natural to our childhood years.

But a look at why we need fun in our lives will help push us in the direction of getting it back.

In each human person are blueprints for living, which we call archetypes. They make up our collective unconscious, so if you are of the species Homo Sapiens, you have inherited them.

One of the major archetypes that each of us has is the child archetype. It is this archetype which "nurtures that part of us that longs to be light-hearted, innocent, and expectant of the wonders of tomorrow. Our child archetype contributes greatly to our ability to continue a sense of playfulness in our lives and to balance the seriousness of adult life." (Carolyn Myss, *Sacred Contracts*).

There is no better time to balance up the child psyche than during our 50-90 growth period. We are the perfect age. We are ready. Often fun has been too long gone and wants to come back home to stay.

How to set the stage for fun:

-1- Live in the present moment

Being in the now is the key to life. Wisdom says there is only now…we have this moment only…attend to it. Place your attention here, not on the past and not on the future, but on this moment.

If we do this we will be well. Our mind will be free of anxiety and worry because no matter what is out of order, no matter what world is crashing around us, in this one single moment everything is well.

And our body is well when our mind is well. It knows innately that no matter what is happening, at our core we are stable and safe.

For most of us this is not what we have practiced in

the past, but it is the natural response of the child.

A teddy bear or a treat can transform a child's heart-wrenching sobs into smiles and even laughter. Police stations and hospitals know this and so do clowns who visit pediatric units.

If you can't remember what it felt like to be a child it is easy enough to find one to observe.

To the child you are observing, there is only now; disbelief is suspended; magic is expected and "let's pretend" is as easy as breathing.

Our human reality is that this single moment is all we have. We know this and now is the time to live it. Living fully in the moment means to be giving complete attention to it.

So as I write these lines I am aware of
-a- what I am feeling, which is full of joy to be

doing what I love; how my body feels, which is slightly strained because I just noticed that my chair is not exactly in alignment with my keyboard; how my mind feels, which is clear and refreshed because it is mid-morning (my best writing time);

-b- what I am smelling, which is the incense I burned last night;

-c- what I am hearing, which is the silence I need in which to do my best work;

-d- what I am seeing, which, beside my computer screen, is the tree outside my window being blown by a semi-hurricane wind.

My challenge is to stay focused on this moment only and not on the day's to-do list, or on the amount of time I'm spending at the computer, or on the next chapter waiting to be written.

When we are in the moment, our minds are no longer in overdrive. And minds not in overdrive are free to play.

Minds not in overdrive are free to see the beauty in the moment.

Minds not in overdrive are free to steep themselves in their natural capacity for delight.

And "the quality of life is in proportion, always, to the capacity for delight". (Julia Cameron, *The Artist's Way*).

When we are centered on the moment that we are in, we are connected to ourselves. Being connected to ourselves is our deep need, and the quality of our life depends on it.

-2- Doing it the easy way

They say there are two ways to do something, either the hard way or the easy way. It is interesting to check out your belief about this.

For many years I acted on the belief that the hard

way was the superior way. The harder it was to do, the more worthwhile it was. I seemed to be telling myself that the degree of value depended on the level of complication, sweat, and stress involved. One thing was certain, the hard way guaranteed a minimum of fun.

But then I read this line by Deepak Chopra: "…the Universe (Spirit) arranges the easy way out of love for us". It has become my mantra.

Now my first question, in every situation, is "What is the easy way through this?" It is another way of asking, "How can I inject some fun into this big, serious job I'm lining up?" Because fun in equals stress out.

For example, I have been exploring an ancient personality indicator tool called the Enneagram. The Enneagram depicts nine major personality types, which it numbers accordingly.

I am a number One. According to the authors of

What's My Type:The Enneagram System, the type One personality has an addiction to perfection, is compulsive, buries anger, and needs to develop strength and forbearance.

A rather heavy diagnosis, I thought.

But reading on, I found this wonderful line, "(for the One)…deepening the pleasures of sexuality is a way to allow a wider awareness and a more playful self to emerge". Now that sounds better. It appears that one way I can overhaul my personality is to have sex.

How's that for discovering the easy way to achieve my ideal personality.

Another how-to-do-it-the-easy-way discovery involves books.
I live in a small center so if a particular book isn't on the modestly stocked shelves of our local bookstore, the special order process, taking an average of two months, or purchasing over the Internet is the only option.

However, I find the biggest drawback is this. When the book finally arrives, it may or may not live up to my expectations.

But now we have the phenomenon (in larger centers, of course) of the come on in, stay all day if you want, and read anything on our shelves bookstores. They have become reason enough for a trip. I thought it was a brilliant touch that most of them housed a coffee bar, until I found one with a restaurant that offered lunch and homemade sweets, and was licensed for beer and wine.

Scores of readers fill this modern version of a bookstore.

Two and three stories high, serviced by escalators, and often providing overstuffed chairs, these stores invite the buyer to browse, read, study, take notes, or inspect any book on any shelf, and all of them brand new.

I spend hours that pass like seconds. And the bonus

of all bonuses, when I finally make a selection, I know exactly what I am buying.

Then there is the fun of reading itself. Someone said, to be able to learn is to be young, and whoever keeps the joy of learning fresh is forever young.

Joy of learning

There are many easy ways to learn something new everyday.

I recently watched my one-year-old grandchild, Aidan, and realized that a young child is engaged in learning in every waking moment. He never ceases to be on the job.

He studies every face around him; he explores every object he encounters (primarily by giving it the taste test); he learns different textures as he crawls over them, both indoors and out; he experiments with tastes at every meal.

And he has no problem figuring out the easiest way through. When his first trip over a mat outside my front door proved too scratchy on his knees, next trip he simply made a sharp left and crawled around it.

For him, just to be awake is to experience the joy of learning.

Opportunities for fun and fresh learning are all around us older children, too.

There are the traditional ways, such as, read and study, watch documentaries, attend library-sponsored seminars and information days, hang out in museums and art galleries.

>Or if you want to update you can
>-a- listen to your adult children describe their workplace or their lifestyle
>-b- let your grandchildren show you how to use their high-tech toys

-c- experiment with new ways to do an old hobby

-d- volunteer for something you are passionate about

-e- shop on line, join a chat room, date (you're the right age)

-f- get a body part pierced

-g- join Toastmasters and conquer your fear of public speaking

How easy any of these undertakings will be depends solely on what mindset you bring to it.

Come to the starting line resolved to find the easy way through, and you will. With a whole lot of fun thrown in as a bonus.

-3- Be spontaneous

It was my last day in Australia. I had come to the end of my visit but I had some unfinished business. I had not yet gone into the green, sparkling ocean. It was still spring and the water temperature left a bit to be desired.

On my way home from shopping I decided to stop at the beach, which is located in the middle of the shopping district because the city is on the waterfront.

Disappointed to be leaving without connecting in a physical way with this beautiful landscape, I waded, ankle-deep, into the water. Taking my time, I gradually waded to knee level. Not so cold.

I stood another while. The sun was glorious. The sand was warm. The water called me to it, and I responded, clothes and all.

I romped and played and made a life-time memory.

In between splashes I overheard a man on the beach ask his wife, "Does that woman know she has all her clothes on?"

At Our Age

That woman did, and that woman also knew that she was having a great deal of fun.

Celebration is another way to be spontaneous. Celebrating is important because it acknowledges life. In fact, we hurt when we don't have anyone to share the significance of major events in our lives, like the ninety-second birthday of my beloved Aunt, and the birth of my third grandchild, both happening this month.

Our lives are filled with reasons for celebration. Take this one, for example.

It was an especially sunny and warm afternoon for Canadian maritime climes, given the late fall date of October 31st.

The community walking track where I was "doing my daily" is located next to a school. My attention was suddenly grabbed by a fun-loving (yes, adult) voice on the school's public address system with its outside speakers engaged for the occasion, which proceeded to brightly say, "Alright ghosts and goblins, time to line up for #9 school bus."

The voice was then followed by the music and lyrics of "Ghostbusters", "Do the Monster Mash", and "One eyed Purple People Eater".

Anyone within earshot couldn't help but feel the delight that spilled over from the Halloween celebrations going on deep within the secret halls of the school and out into the surrounding neighborhood.

Gratitude Notebook

Get a small notebook and at the end of each day, write one positive aspect that it held.

Or write five things you are thankful for in the day. These may be infinitely miniscule or gargantuan.

At Our Age

What happens when you do this is quite lovely. Your mind and heart release their spontaneous delight at life.

Everything becomes a cause for celebration, from winning the lotto to finding a dime. An attitude of celebration throws the doors of opportunity open and draws more of our good to us.

Spontaneity releases solutions to problems, new insights, and answers we have been waiting a long time to find.

A friend just reminded me of her favorite lyrics from a song by Jon Bon Jovi and they go something like this, "we go around all dressed in black, as serious as a heart attack".

That's what we adults do, and a heart attack is often what we get.

Let's quit doing that. It takes only the tiniest shift of focus, barely a centimeter, not even a half inch, to form the "don't take it all so seriously" mindset.

Look for the "how to turn this into fun" opening in whatever you are doing and feeling. It's right there waiting to break in on you, maybe something as easy as telling a good joke.

Have you heard this one?

"A Third Age couple got married. Every night, after getting into bed, the new bride took a large pill.

Unable to contain his curiosity any longer, the new groom finally asked her why. He was immediately informed that it was her youth pill and that she took it to keep young.

Hmm. No, he couldn't resist. He waited till his youthful bride was asleep, stealthily located the magic pills and swallowed three of them.

In the morning, upon awakening, the bride found herself alone.

Her groom was not in bed, not anywhere upstairs, not anywhere downstairs.

Finally she located him sitting outside their front yard, on the curb, sobbing.

"John, John, what ever is the matter?"

Through heart-rending sobs she heard, "I missed the sch… sch…ool b…bus."

RESOURCES

The Deeper Wound. Deepak Chopra, Harmony Books, New York. 2001.

Sacred Contracts. Carolyn Myss, Random House, New York, NY. 2001

Toni Smart of **Smart Actions**, Archetype Consultant.

Phone: 011 61 7 3876 2442 email: smartactions@optusnet.com.au

The Power of Now. Eckhart Tolle. Namaste Publishing, Vancouver, BC. 1997.

Chapter Five
At the Ready

The heart at any age can fall in love.

You may never have been in love with another human being, although that is unlikely, but you definitely have been in love. You have felt, at some time in your life, enamoured of something.

As a child it might have been a pet, your family, your bike, your stuffed animal, or your imaginary friend; it might have been Christmas, the zoo, the farm, your grandparents' house, a special book.

As an adolescent it was that teen idol (or several), a star athlete, a Hollywood actor/actress, a teacher or a coach. It might have been playing a sport at which you excelled, a particular movie (one friend says he is still in love with Debbie Reynolds ever since her role as Tammy), a dream or a life goal.

And then, for at least some of us, there was that first girl or guy who made you fumble and babble and unable to breathe.

Most of us have a memory of being starry-eyed and breathless over something. And if your memory tells you that nothing felt better, it is telling you right.

Nothing feels better than being alive at the core of your being.

Nothing exhilarates like the feeling that you can do or be anything.

Nothing scintillates like every neutron and electron in every cell of your body tingling and dancing and sparking with possibility. No wonder we do it, fall in love, that is.

Even though a sexual expression of the experience of falling in love is perhaps the most intense form of expression—-and amen to that —- we can have an "I'm in love experience" all the time. In fact, that's the key, according to Laura Day in *Practical Intuition in Love*.

Being in love before you fall in love, says Day, is what we have to do. And she is right because an immutable Law of the Universe is that like attracts like.

Well, now. Just exactly what are we saying? We are saying that if you want to attract a lover you need to already be in love.

Right about now you might be asking how you are supposed to manage this… this being in love before you fall in love.

You will love Day's answer, it is this: you need simply to be in a state of pleasure. That's it. Create pleasure in every moment. No matter what the moment is, easy or difficult, put some aspect of pleasure in it. Here is the reason why.

Our chemistry mechanisms are akin to those of every other member of the animal kingdom, and the underlying law is that chemistry responds to chemistry.

When we are in love, our body chemistry changes. Hormone and chemical levels are accelerated.

You can easily recall how that state felt (right?), nothing less than wonderful.

The point to make is that when we experience pleasure, our bodies produce the same chemical changes as falling in love does. So in order to have our body chemistry

At Our Age

always at the ready, we need simply to always be in pleasure mode.

We need to be having and being and doing what feels good. In fact, the endorphins like serotonin and oxytocin that pleasure produces in us are often called the feel-good hormones.

Serotonin calms anxiety and improves mood. It affects our appetites, sexual and otherwise.

Oxytocin is involved in any aspect of love and is called the love hormone. It is secreted by a structure of the brain called the hypothalamus, and released into the bloodstream in pleasure-producing circumstances.

For example, when we share a pleasant meal with others, we increase our level of oxytocin. The increased hormone tells our mind that all is very well. We relax. We are in re-creation mode.

Then there are our pheromones.

Pheromones are the mysteries of odor in human sexuality. It has become crystal clear to scientists that human pheromones affect us more than most people can imagine.

We are surprised to be told that chemical communication, specifically, what we smell, is more important to sexual behavior than what we see, hear or touch.

Scientist's have also shown that male human pheromones trigger a subconscious sexual response in women. Pheromones are odorless and consciously undetectable to the human nose, but because women have a naturally better defined sense of smell they subconsciously pick up male human pheromones right away and become instantly sexually attracted to the wearer or the bearer of them.

So it is not surprising that androstenone, a male human pheromone, has been packaged and is for sale. See www.pheromones.com.

One of the ads at that website totes this info:

"Ever meet someone and feel this unbelievable chemistry? Doesn't happen very often, but these are pheromones at work. Send out that pheromone chemical message of sex to women and they will crave you, desire you and want to get to know you….". Very interesting.

Our chemical response to pleasure is important because these hormones tell our mind and emotions and body, that in this one moment our world is perfect, that all is as it should be, and that we are beautiful.

And then all that is beautiful and all that should be begins to move toward us. That is the Law of Attraction, the first law of the Universe, in operation.

But back to the job at hand, which is a consideration of this task: how to create the "I'm in love" hormones that will turn you into a love magnet before you are in love, so you can draw the love of your life to you or recharge the one you already have, the one whose battery is running low.

Step #1. Make a Pleasure List.

What do you have fun doing? What do you love doing? What makes you feel wonderful? What makes you feel delightful? Make a list of the big and the small.

On my list are reading, walking, dancing, skating, phone chats with my adult far-away children, protecting my health, writing love letters, seminars on cutting-edge thinking, sharing a confidence with a trusted friend, slow mornings, getting and giving compliments, crocus and daffodils coming up through the snow, a self-care day, sending care packages, the night sky, hearing real-life love stories, my morning pages.

It's a list that is organic, as they say, which means it is always changing and growing. Make a large and thorough list. Include the new and daring.

Step #2. Do something from Step #1 every day.

Step #3. Pleasure the moment.

Slow down and taste, see, touch, smell, speak pleasure.

What do you need to do in the moment to feel good? What do you need to change about the moment in order to feel good? You can change something, even some very small thing about the worse situation.

Drudgery can be combated.

For example, you have to wait two hours in a doctor's office.

Put pleasure in it by reading a book that you keep in the car for just such an opportunity, do your muscle-relaxing routine or your Kegel exercises, rest, listen to favorite tapes/CD's on your walkman, enjoy the social aspect of the situation, meditate, write a letter, make a to-do list, organize your handbag or houseclean your wallet (if that gives you pleasure), pray for world peace or your loved ones, anticipate a good medical outcome from your visit, etc. In fact in two hours you can do just about all of the above…

At every moment, ask, "What can I do to love/pleasure myself at this moment?" Then answer it.

There is always some small pleasure you can introduce, no matter where you are:
- a - You can forge a smile onto your tight face and hold it for sixty seconds. Feel the change it makes to your tense body and mind.
- b - You can breathe in from your abdomen for a count of four, hold for a count of four and breathe out for a count of eight. Do this a few times and feel your whole body relax.
- c - You can drink water. Water re-hydrates brain cells immediately.
- d - You can set aside an hour a week for a date

with yourself. Just you and yourself doing something you love to do. Having a love-in.

Be in love with your own company.

Set a weekly date to celebrate being alone with yourself. It is in that space that you will discover what you truly love and how to truly pleasure yourself.

It is really only then that we can teach another how to pleasure us, sexually, socially, and intellectually.

What to do about loneliness

Speaking of a date for one, this might be a good time to talk about loneliness.

I have been living alone for about a year and a half and it continues to be a formidable challenge.

For the first few months it was easy. I had just exited a world where I had been a twenty-four hour caregiver, so having no one but me to be responsible for was almost a natural high.

But as time passed, evenings began to weigh heavy and weekends became downright foreboding.

I had two choices. I could look for ways to escape the pain, or I could learn how to handle life on my own. I chose the latter because I knew that once I learned how to be my own source, I would no longer need to fear anything else life could hand me.

That was the freedom I sought and the freedom I continue to work at acquiring. It is an ongoing process.

Oriah Mountain Dreamer writes these penetrating lines: "I want to know if you can be alone with yourself and if you like the company you keep in the empty moments."

This is an empowering goal. When being alone no

longer frightens or cripples you, when you can laugh at the empty moments, you are free.

And here's the best part. When you are free, your ideal lover will not be able to resist the magnetism of your freedom.

Empty moments

Here is what I am learning about handling a surplus of empty moments:

#1. Do not fear them

Instead, relax into them. That's right. Relax into them. Just be in them, as if it is all right that they are there. Just let them be.

Author Natalie Goldberg, in her book, *Wild Mind,* tells a story about her spiritual director, Kagiri Roshi.

She had complained to him about the loneliness of her life as a writer. When she asked him if he was ever lonely he replied that yes, he was, but that it was only loneliness and he didn't let it "toss him away".

Do not let the empty places toss you away.

Tomorrow, when you are only a day or two away from the weekend and you tense with the dread of being swallowed up by its empty places, take a moment and do this.

Put your arms around that thought. Hold it gently, right there, next to you. Allow it to be with you. It is an important part of you, not an enemy. Welcome it and receive the gift it has for you.

If you do that, what you will discover is that it will no longer terrify you.

Instead it will change itself into an ally, into a new feeling called courage. Into strength. Into thriving.

Kiss the frog and release its beauty.

#2. Proceed as if

Become aware of what you are thinking.

What do you want instead of the empty places?

Be clear and specific; describe it in detail for yourself. Let yourself feel the way you will feel when what you want will actually appear in your life.

What you are doing is "proceeding as if".

You are feeling and thinking as if you already have what you are asking for. You are focusing on what you want and not on what you don't have. This is a very powerful practice. Where you put your focus is very important.

These lines from a Sesame Street song have great wisdom in them, "where you put your eyes, that's about the size, that's about the size of it."

The puppet lesson is about perspective. Live from the space you want to be in emotionally, not the space you are in.

Put the eyes of your mind on what you know is on its way to you. If you do this for only a few moments at a time, a few times a day, you are making enormous progress.

You are creating the life you want. Your desired outcome will appear in your life with perfect timing.

#3. Make Plans

Line up something for an evening or two during the week, and for at least one day on the weekend.

I am finding that one planned activity here and there eases the strain a great deal and initiates a flow.

At Our Age

One of my friends lost her husband recently. She reports that her days are becoming easier now that she realizes she was expecting others to create a new life for her and has since stepped up to the plate herself. She has become her own initiator. Be your own initiator and the Universe will rush in to meet you.

Being in love is a perspective that gives unspeakable power to our living.

Start your day as if you are in love.

Walk as if you are in love.

Work as if you are in love.

Relate to everyone, co-workers, neighbours, in-laws, grocery store staff etc. as if you are in love.

See the landscape and seascape and skyscape as if you are in love.

Remember, thoughts are electro-magnetic energy. Emotions are electro-magnetic energy. They draw/create in kind.

When you are filled with a sense of awe you create awe in the outward circumstances of your life. If you think and feel gratitude (a natural response when we are in love), you set the Universe free to create more of what you are grateful for.

My twenty-something niece recently decided she is ready for a serious relationship and wanted to know how to begin finding her ideal partner. This is what she needs to do.

Her first step is to get very clear on what she wants in a lover.

Yes, make a list, again. Get it outside your head and on paper.

What are the qualities your partner must have? Ask yourself what you value most in a partner at this time in your life.

Is it emotional maturity? Financial security? Shared interests/goals? High-priority sex life? Is geographical location an issue?

An easy way to know what you want is to ask yourself what you don't want.

For example, "I don't want a partner who depends on me for emotional security" becomes "I want a partner who is strong enough emotionally to face life alone if he/she has to."

Ask what is most important to you and also ask in what areas you are willing to compromise.

Be as clear as you can about what you are looking for.

Her second step is to work on herself.

That's right. I heard someone say that if you had faulty parenting, become the parent you didn't have.

Well, basically you will attract the lover you want when you become the lover you want.

Self-knowledge is absolutely critical in all our relationships.

The good news is that at our age we have already garnered a substantial amount. That is one of the perks.

The Myers Briggs Personality Type Indicator and the Enneagram are two tools to turn you into an expert on your own personality. So is the study of your Archetypes.

There has been no greater breakthrough for me than to discover, through these effective instruments for self-knowledge, the limitations of some of the beliefs I have been carrying around, and operating out of, for many, many years.

We pick up beliefs about ourselves from infancy on.

We do not taste freedom, the fullness of being adult, until we begin to examine these beliefs in the light of our own wisdom, to question their validity, and to abandon them if they are found wanting.

On one occasion I casually remarked to my Life Coach that I was no good at anything technological (such as computers). His instant reply was, "How do you know that?"

I was pulled up short. How did I know that?

Well, I think it's a childhood conclusion I made about fifty years ago, and I no longer remember why. But I locked it in, and in doing so I locked out all potential.

With that insight, I bravely signed up for a beginner's computer class, and have since launched a career that relies heavily on the remarkable capabilities of computer technology.

So an important part of self-knowledge is figuring out where you may have been gypping yourself. Who told you that you couldn't _____. Fill in the blank.

Who told you that you couldn't fall in love at your age?

Take this "preparing for my perfect partner time" and spend it on you.

Put your focus on discovering who you are and who you can easily become.

Do not use the past as the measuring stick for who you can be now, or for the future you can create. That is a common mistake we all make.

Who you were is not all you can be. Stop telling yourself it is too late. It is never too late to become who you want to be.

Age is an illusion, don't buy into it.

Don't speak limiting words, they usually start with, "I can't…"

Don't think limiting thoughts, our thoughts become our reality.

Think unlimited possibility. Study yourself. Renowned author Deepak Chopra says, "Don't work on your relationship. Work on yourself."

Create yourself. Love yourself. Date yourself. Nurture yourself. Pleasure yourself. Then you will draw the perfect partner to you, or re-create the relationship you already have.

RESOURCES

The Secret of Eros: Mysteries in Human Sexuality. James Kohl and Robert Francoeur. 2002.

What's My Type? Kathleen Hurley and Theodore Dobson, HarperSanFrancisco, NY. 1991. (Studies in the Enneagram).

Practical Intuition in Love. Laura Day, HarperPerennial, USA. 1998.

Myers Briggs Personality Type Indicator available at **www.discoveryourpersonality.com/MBTI.html**

Enneagram
www.9types.com

Chapter Six
Sex – At Our Age?

In sex is hidden a door to infinity. Open it.
David and Ellen Ramsdale

A white-haired man was standing onshore leisurely casting his line into the crystal sun-soaked waters of his favorite fishing spot when he heard a voice say, "How do you do?"

His search revealed the source of the voice to be a frog perched at his feet.

"Well, well now," he replied. "Look at that. In all my eighty years I have never seen a talking frog."

"Actually," said the frog, "I am a very beautiful

woman and if you will kiss me and release me I will grant your wildest sexual fantasy".

"Really!" said the man.

"Most certainly," said the frog.

The man then proceeded to scoop the frog into his shirt pocket, pack up his gear, and head for home.

"Stop! Stop!" cried the frog. "What are you doing? I told you I would grant your wildest sexual fantasy and all you have to do is kiss me."

Hesitating, but only a moment, the fisherman replied,

"Well, it's a bit like this. At my age I'd rather have a talking frog."

If you agree with the man, you should probably just go on to the next chapter. If not, let's go right to the bottom line:

Sex is good. It helps us live longer and these are the reasons why.

Physical Benefits:

Sex is an aerobic exercise that induces deep breathing and accelerated heart rate.

It sends blood rushing throughout the body (otherwise known as good circulation) and especially to the genitals, keeping important muscles strong and producing in them a state of health. And our genital muscles are not the muscles we want to let atrophy.

Sexual exercise boosts energy, acts as a time out, and even strengthens not only muscle tissue, but bone tissue as well.

It increases our testosterone level, and that is good news because testosterone is necessary for the sexual health of both men and women.

And did you know that the experts now assure us that sex reduces pain? That's right.

So all this time we could not only have been saying yes, tonight, dear, because I have a headache.

We also could have been healing ourselves a whole lot easier and faster, and playing all the while.

Emotional Benefits:

As with any exercise, sexual activity releases beta-endorphin, a natural body substance that is hundreds of times more powerful than morphine.

This release begins just twelve minutes into a workout, which is a very good reason for prolonging the activity.

Beta-endorphins alter our emotional state from negative to positive, from worry and stress to love and other positive emotions.

They reduce our pain level, and stimulate memory retention and learning ability. Acupuncture is an endorphin-related technique.

And here's a by-product not to be sneezed at, because of its emotional benefits sex can ward off disease.

Seratonin, another natural body chemical, is also released. Seratonin acts on the central nervous system and produces feelings of well being, a heightened spirit, and reduced depression.

It is also known as the brain's painkiller. It produces that all-important "I am happy" feeling, calms anxiety, and induces sleep.

These natural drugs are produced by the glands and carried to the brain and nervous system by the blood. You can see how sexual activity facilitates their production.

Spiritual Benefits:

Considering the spiritual benefits of sex is the same as considering the spiritual benefits of play. Not something we have often thought about, but when we do, there they are.

Sex is play. But what is play?

Play is the activity of the soul, our inner creator being allowed out.

Therefore sex, too, is the inner creator being allowed out and it is play par excellence. We always need play, at any age, because when we play we are, for a few brief moments, taken completely out of ourselves.

And that is what ecstasy is. Play takes us to ecstasy. But where do we go when we are "out of ourselves"?

When you sit in the audience in Carnegie Hall or

in the great opera houses of Europe and feel transported by the beauty of the performance, to where are you transported?

Well, the answer to that question is the whole point about sex.

The answer is, you are carried into a brief moment of union with infinity, with the mystical, with the divine.

It's not so much that we are carried out of ourselves as that we are carried into the truest part of ourselves, to our core, where the deepest wellspring of life is. And sex does that.

When we experience orgasm in sexual play, we experience ecstasy.

Orgasm is an ecstatic state. Ecstasy is ecstasy is ecstasy whether its source has been a sexual orgasm or a deep meditation.

Whether it is the saint seeking oneness with the Divine through meditation or a lover seeking oneness with the beloved through love-making, the sexual desire is the longing of the spirit and soul for ecstasy, that is, for oneness with the Infinite.

Sexuality and Spirituality

Perhaps linking sex and spirituality is a stretch for you, a new concept.

Perhaps you have spent a lifetime believing that sex and soul are polar opposites. Enemies, even.

That is my sexual saga. I have been trained, taught, and conditioned in a sex education that was based on a totally erroneous premise.

That premise is that the human person is divided into two separate parts, the body and the soul.

At Our Age

The soul is superior and the body is inferior. Sexuality belongs to the body. It needs to be controlled, reigned in, used sparingly, and carefully guarded lest unbridled pleasure prevail.

We are familiar with the results of this doctrine of sexual repression. They are guilt, shame, denial, and sexual perversion.

So a very important part of my third Age growth has been to question the script for my sexuality that I not only inherited but that I have accepted, unquestioned, for far too many years. I am re-writing the script.

My new script looks like this.

"Never repress sex. Never be against it. Rather, go deeply into it.... with great love. Go like an explorer. Search all the nooks and crannies of your sexuality and you will stumble upon your spirituality. Then you will become free. The future will have a totally different vision of sex for you…more fun, more joy, more friendship, more play…" Osho Rajneesh.

As humans we have a deep capacity for the mystical.

We know that to be completely taken out of ourselves feels natural. We naturally seek a "high". That is the allure of alcohol and drugs.

We are at home in the realm of the mystical, in the realm of the ecstatic.

Orgasm is a natural door to that ecstasy. And ecstasy is ecstasy.

Whether it is two people taking each other there or one woman/man taking herself/himself there, sexuality is our deep core.

Where is the room for shame or guilt? Our capacity

for orgasm is a gift, given to us by an Infinite Intelligence for our utmost good.

Far from being the cause of the separation of body and soul, sex, to the contrary, is a powerful tool for uniting our human personality, for integrating all the parts of ourselves, and for healing the deep interior rift that many of us have carried since childhood.

If you are experiencing some shock or hesitation or any form of discomfort at what you are reading here, gently absorb it and give it some reflection. Yes, you can dare to believe that sex is deeply wholesome and deeply spiritual.

Tantric Sex

The Tantric understanding of the spiritual power of sex is not new. The Eastern traditions are now revealing and teaching the Western world the sexual wisdom which they have possessed for centuries.

Tantra is a body of writing/doctrine that contains Buddhist mystical teachings and ritual.

The basic teaching of Tantra is that everything is permeated with God, or the Divine. Orgasmic surrender is understood as a melting and merging into the Divine.

For the practitioner of Tantric Sex, the result of sex is to become aligned with our sacred Self.

Eastern Tantras have always viewed sex as a pathway to higher consciousness.

The word Tantra is Sanskrit, the sacred language of Hinduism, and means to expand or extend.

The practice of Tantric techniques is not only celebrated as a way to expand and extend our level of conscious awareness during lovemaking.

It is also recognized by modern day science for the

positive medical results it produces.

Tantric sexual positions are considered to be more physically stimulating, especially for women.

This may be because intimacy is a key ingredient of Tantric sex, a primary focus.

Sexual intimacy is a closeness and a communication level that surpasses the level of physical communication.

Sometimes we speak about having a spiritual connection with someone, or about finding a soul mate.

For many lovers, perhaps for women more than for men, intimacy needs to be present in order for passion to get ignited. The soul connection is the turn on and then the body follows suit.

This is the Tantric approach. The experts at Tantra at Tahoe (www.tantraattahoe.com) say, "Your body becomes ecstatic when it gets in tune with your spirit."

And the best news of all is, there is no age limit. In fact, the gentle approach of Tantric sex is particularly suited to the not-as-young-as-it-used-to-be body.

Give your sex life a makeover. Explore Tantric sex. (More information at the end of this chapter).

Sex For One (book by Betty Dodson)

Validating "sex for one" may be a quantum leap for you.

There's a good chance that a major part of your script, probably several chapters of it, has been devoted to the "M" word. The word masturbation probably conjures up more immediate shame than any other sexually related term.

The first book to rescue me from deep sexual woundedness was *Sexual Energy Ecstacy* by Ellen and David Ramsdale.

Through it I was given new eyes and a new heart for the miraculous human experience we have labeled "masturbation", or worse, "self-abuse".

The Ramsdales have a better word, which is, "self-loving".

It is a term they borrowed from Betty Dodson in her book, *Sex For One: The Joy of Self-loving*. They maintain that our historical guilt and shame is not about sex itself but about the attitude we have inherited.

They go on to say, "As a private, uninhibited opportunity to explore the sexual and sensual potential of your own body, the positive power of self-loving actually opens you up to being a better…partner when in bed with another."(Ramsdale p.95).

Examine your sexual beliefs.

Search your heart to find out if they resonate with your own deep knowing or are they an inheritance which, as a mature adult, you have never examined, and which no longer fit who you have become.

Not having a partner does not mean you cannot have the important and unequalled benefits of sex.

A seventy-two year old man asked Dr. Sandor Gardos, Clinical Sexologist, the following question:

" I'm 72 and I still masturbate. My wife died about a year ago and I now masturbate more often than ever (about three to four times a week). Is this normal?"

This was the answer he received:

"Absolutely! Not only is it normal, but it is actually good for you! Although sometimes people are under the mistaken notion that sexuality is somehow reserved for the young, in reality, sexuality is part of all of us. There is nothing wrong with masturbating at any age. In fact, studies show that, barring serious health conditions, rates of masturbation do not really decline until people reach their 90's…it is downright healthy! It has been speculated that frequent ejaculations can help keep the prostate healthy, which becomes more of a concern as men become older. So my advice is: Keep it up!"

Betty Dodson's book, *Sex for One*, has an important purpose: to liberate us, and women in particular.

The statistics on the number of women who spend years having sex without the experience of orgasm are heartbreaking. This story is an example.

A friend and I attended a seminar on menopause. Good for us.

One of the presenters, a sex therapist, engaged the group in open and graphic discussion about the sex act "at our age".

Another thing she did was to lead us, amid shyness, self-consciousness and eventually some good laughs, through the Kegel exercises, several levels of Kegel exercises, to be exact.

The Kegel exercises are designed to tighten male and female sexual muscles and heighten our capacity for orgasm.

At the end of the presentation, my friend, married for many years and the mother of four adult children, fell silent. Then she turned to me with deep sadness in her face and voice.

"You know what I just learned?" she asked. "I've never had an orgasm".

Is this story a rare occurrence? No. It isn't. That's why Dodson's work, books, seminars, and lectures are dedicated to changing it.

And self-loving is where orgasmic success begins.

Sexuality and Disability

If mental or physical disability is not part of your world or part of a loved one's world, you probably have not given much thought to the topic of sex in the life of the mentally or physically challenged.

But if your sex life is affected in any way by something as commonplace as arthritis, you may want to read on.

According to Dr. Linda Mona, nationally recognized expert and advocate for raising disabled sexuality awareness, sex is even more important to the lives of the disabled than to the abled.

Because of the handicap, loss of identity can be severe; the sense of womanhood or manhood is already decimated. It is only successful sexual experience that can restore that.

In Denmark, the government is leading the way in experimenting with solutions to this important aspect of the life of a mentally or physically challenged person.

Government funding is currently provided for escort services for the handicapped.

I'll give you a moment to go back and read that last sentence again.

For example, twice a month one mentally challenged middle-aged man with the mental capacity of a five-year old is accompanied by his social worker to an escort service where he receives sex.

The results are encouraging. He no longer preys on women and is able to maintain a more stable daily life.

Another example is a man with very little mobility

in any part of his body due to cerebral palsy.

But his sex drive is still very alive and well. And so is his brain.

He has become his own advocate for his sexual needs, and now receives government funded escort service in his home once a month.

Of course my intention here is not to oppose or defend the morality of any particular sexual practice; that is the focus of another book.

My intention is to promote the value of sex for humanity.

For important education on this topic go to www.mypleasure.com. Click on Education and then Sex & Disability.

This site is a complete resource for education, information and sexual products for people with disabilities.

Topics include reduced mobility due to arthritis, multiple sclerosis, cerebral palsy, muscular dystrophy, and spinal cord injury.

Products that help include:

- items that are easy to put on and take off
- items that operate with limited physical movement
- items that extend one's reach
- remote controls
- longer handles
- items that can be configured into multiple positions for easy-reach access.

Other products are specifically designed for:

- sensory and nerve impairments
- erection or penile difficulties

- bowel and bladder issues
- women's needs
- special concerns items which are described as "items which present solutions in life".

Sex is your gift.

Sex is your door to infinity.

There is no age limit on personal growth or on whole-person living.

Whatever your age you are the right age to listen to your inner being, to examine the script that has been written there, and to re-write it for yourself.

No area of human experience requires this more than our sexuality.

Whether you have a partner or not, whether you are making love with another or with yourself, "love is the fragrance that proves that the one-thousand petalled lotus in the innermost core of your being has bloomed". Osho Rajneesh

RESOURCES

Sex For One: The Joy of Self-Loving. Betty Dodson. Three Rivers Press, New York. 1996

Sexual Energy Ecstasy: A Practical Guide to Lovemaking Secrets of the East and West. David and Ellen Ramsdale. Bantam Books, USA. 1993

The Vagina Monologues. Eve Ensler. Villard, New York. 2001

The Unhealed Wound: the Church and Human Sexuality. Eugene Kennedy. St. Martin's Griffen, New York. 2001

The Soul of Sex: Cultivating Life as an Act of Love. Thomas Moore. HarperPerennial. 1998.

<u>Sex For Life: The Lover's Guide to Male Sexuality</u>. David Saul, MD. Apple Publishing, Vancouver, BC.

Any book by Margot Anand. She is known as the mother of Tantra.

www.margotanand.com

www.mypleasure.com

Chapter Seven
Getting the Money You Want

I'm rich beyond my wildest dreams, I am, I am, I am.
Tom and Penelope Pauley

I have no financial expertise so this chapter will not offer any professional advice on how to manage money.

Instead I'd like to tell you about the prosperity theory which I have recently begun to set in motion in my financial life.

This theory is based on the premise that abundance is our natural birthright, that abundance is the natural condition of the Universe and that the Universe, as we know, deals in trillions of trillions of everything.

Consider the statistics: our galaxy, the Milky Way, has two billion stars in it (the sun is one of them).

The diameter of this galaxy is a hundred thousand light years.

The nearest galaxy to ours is two and a half million light years away; it belongs to our Local Group, which has more than thirty galaxies in it.

The number of groups in the Universe at this point in our evolution is immeasurable.

We can be at home with the concept of abundance.

In order to create abundance in our finances our first consideration is not how to better balance the budget or how to make surefire investments.

Our first consideration is a more unlikely one, the consideration of our personal attitude toward money.

That's right. Wealth is an inside job. Your underlying belief about money is affecting your dough flow.

You may not be aware of your money beliefs, but you have them.

Some of these may sound familiar:

"There's never enough to go around"

"Money isn't spiritual"

"The rich are suspect"

"It wouldn't be right to charge what I'm worth"

"I'd have more money if I could just get a break"

"What can you expect in this economy"

"There are a lot of things more important than money"

"Everything is so expensive"

"It is so hard to save money"

And the number one block to acquiring money, "I don't deserve to have a lot of money".

Low self-esteem, our 'I don't deserve' belief, is the number one issue for all of us.

Statistics record a whopping 90% for the tally on the portion of the population suffering from low self-esteem, and it overflows into and negatively impacts our finances.

So where do we begin discovering how to get the money we want?

We begin by changing our money beliefs.

Beliefs are what we get when we think a thought over and over, so we can get new beliefs the same way we got the old ones. We think new thoughts, and we do it over and over.

Let's start by refreshing our minds about why everything hinges on our thoughts.

The quote at the beginning of this chapter is actually the title of a book, *I'm Rich Beyond My Wildest Dreams, I am, I am, I am* by Tom Pauley and his daughter, Penelope Pauley. The book is based on a natural law of the universe called the Law of Attraction.

The Law of Attraction is a scientific law which operates at the quantum level of creation. I referred to this concept in Chapter One and would like to come back to it now.

Here it is:
All creation is made of electro-magnetic energy. The law of this energy is to attract to itself what is like itself.

We are familiar with magnetic force and understand why our fridge magnets cling to our fridge, providing the fridge is made of the same material as the magnet.

What is key for us in this theory we are exploring is the fact that our thoughts - those same ordinary thoughts we think all day long - are made of this same electro-magnetic energy.

Thoughts are energy and they draw to themselves, they create in kind.

The deduction that follows is that we can create our reality. We can create the life we want to live, and that means we can create the prosperity we need and we do so by deliberate thinking.

Yes, our thoughts have that kind of power.

"Oh if we could realize how to live through our minds", said Godfrey Mowatt.

So now that we have our positive beliefs amplified, let's get down to it.

The absolute first step to financial success is to become aware of what you are saying about money because the words we speak come from the beliefs we have.

Perhaps you feel this is trifling advice and you are frothing at the bit for something concrete, something you can take to the bank, so to speak.

I promise you that becoming aware of how you speak and think about money is the most direct route to getting it.

Here is how to begin to use it for attracting the money you want.

Again, start to notice what you are saying about money, and what you aren't saying but are thinking. Then you can do one or more of the following with the negative thought: (the following suggestions are from "Creating Power" by Karim Hajee. It is an incredibly effective program for launching the life you want and deserve and I highly recommend it. Contact information at end of Chapter).-1- You can just take note of it; simply say, "that was a negative thought". If that is all you do you will be making great strides toward changing your thinking habit.

-2- Or you can note the negative thought and just shift your mind to another topic, a positive thought that doesn't have anything to do with the topic of money.

-3- Or you can note the negative thought and replace it with its opposite. Then "I don't deserve" becomes "I deserve".

Practice saying it and thinking it.

"Money isn't spiritual" becomes "money is necessary in order for me to accomplish good works".

"Rich people are suspect" becomes "rich people are those who unlocked the principles of abundance for themselves and for others".

"There isn't enough to go around" becomes "abundance is all there is".

Another highly effective way to get a new mindset is to list your negative thoughts and concepts. Make a list of your beliefs about money as you uncover them, then write their opposite next to them.

Maybe you write, "I hate paying bills", then you write "I love paying my bills", even though you feel as if you are going to choke when you write it.

But remember, in your new world you have all the money you need to pay your bills, and it is certainly true that we really do love the good things we bought with that charge card, you know, things like the phone and lights and fuel for heat.

But please take note of this, it is key:

You do not have to believe the replacement thought.

Again, you do not have to believe the replacement thought.

You only have to think it, or write it.

You only have to repeat it and before long your conscious mind falls in line. And that's when the results you are aiming for start to show up.

I became my own sleuth, standing in the background and watching my thoughts, where they go, where they hang out, where they're favorite haunts are. And as you might expect, it was a bit of a shock to discover where my mind spends most of its money thoughts…yes, in the lack shack.

You know you're hanging out in the lack shack when you hear yourself thinking or saying "I can't afford to.."; "there's too much month at the end of the money"; "I can't pay my bills"; "the economy is down the tubes"; "I'm really afraid about the future". Etc.

You may want to defend this thinking pattern as "just telling it like it is".

But this is the subtle point that makes all the difference.

Your current lack is a circumstance only; it is not the way it is.

The quantum level of reality is the way it is.

An abundant Universe that never stops creating is the way it is.

The facts and figures in your checkbook are recording a passing event. Limitation is not the way it is.

The Universe's totally limitless source is the way it is.

The primal energy that created the cosmos is still doing that, at this very instant. At the quantum level everything is a renewable resource and lack doesn't exist. That means there is a supply of money available to you greater than you can ever use in one lifetime.

The abundance concept may at first seem impossible to fathom because our minds have formed opposite thought habits, but a belief is just a thought we keep repeating. So for a few minutes everyday try these thoughts on for size:

There is an infinite source of supply.Change your mind and you change your world.

You succeed, that is all you ever do. My being wealthy already exists. "Expect your every need to be met, expect the answer to every problem, expect abundance on every level." Eileen Caddy.

Write them on post-it notes and spread them everywhere.

You will be amazed at how quickly your new mindset will affect your day, your attitude, your mood, and your bank account. The results of this small investment of time and thought-energy are exponential.

Two centuries ago Ralph Waldo Emerson expressed the truth about money this way:

"Money, which represents the prose of life, and which is hardly spoken of in parlors without an apology, is, in its effects and laws, as beautiful as roses."

It would appear that our negative money beliefs have been a long time in the making if, in Emerson's century and before, money was "hardly spoken of in parlors without an apology".

How remarkable that he could crash through the

At Our Age

barriers of polite society to expose the true nature of money as representing 'the prose of life'.

How brilliant that he was familiar with both its effects and its laws, and perceived them to be as "beautiful as roses".

What are the beautiful effects of money?

Seriously, what are they for your personal life? What are they for the nation? What are they for the planet?

Renewal, research, restoration, invention, discovery, exploration, advancement, healing, answers, eradication of poverty and injustice, these are some of the beautiful effects of money.

What are the beautiful laws of money?

The laws of money are the laws of the Universe. They are beautiful because they await activation by you and me.

It is law that we create what we think. Dare to believe that the whole process is as simple as that.

One woman says she was desperate to get above water financially and was ready to try anything that had even the hint of a solution, especially if it was free. So she gave this theory a try.

She began to shift her anxious thought that "I can't pay my bills" to "my bills are easily paid in full every month".

She put that thought in her conscious mind daily.

Yesterday she called to jubilantly announce that she is now out of debt and able to live within her monthly budget, and that she still can hardly believe how effortlessly it all came about.

When she began to change her focus, her mind could open up to possibilities she hadn't been able to consider while in a state of anxiety.

It occurred to her that just maybe her financial institution could help. She was right. Within twenty minutes of walking in the door (without an appointment) her debts were amalgamated and a manageable budget was in place.

Now she is working on her next project, manifesting increased income.

Many books describe this process of causing the money you want to show up in your life, and I have listed several of them in the resources at the end of this chapter.

I'd like to touch on one process that several authors agree on and that is a meditation process, perhaps not the first tool you might have expected.

But it is a logical action when we realize that the source of all abundance is within us at our own deep Center. That's always the starting point.

In *Creating Affluence,* Deepak Chopra begins Chapter One with the fact that affluence is our nature. It is totally natural to us and when we are not in affluence we are not whole.

He assures us that we can go to the same place to create affluence for our lives as the Universe goes to create "a cluster of nebulas, a galaxy of stars, a rain forest, a human body or a thought"(Chopra). This is because we have the universe's true nature, which the author calls the field of all possibilities, or the unified field, within us.

Scientists and quantum physicists confirm the existence of this field, and our relationship to it.

We are a field of all possibilities and an effective way to access that field is through meditation.

A simple method is to find a quiet spot to sit.

Relax your body (drop your shoulders and let the chair or floor or ground support your weight).
Breathe in and out gently without pausing until you

feel a connection to your Center.

Then just be in it.

Release your money needs there, into the field of all possibilities. Receive your abundance.

Know it is flowing to you.

Stay twenty minutes if you can, breathing yourself back into the Center when you feel you have wandered out of it.

Be easy. You only have to open to the flow. It is that easy. It is that uncomplicated.

For example, several months had passed since I had loaned money to someone, and I realized that I had formed a defeatist mindset about recovering it. Within days of my working on changing the mindset through meditation, the money showed up.

Here is a summary of the steps to take to get the money you want:

-1- observe your beliefs about money

-2- think/write the opposite of the negative beliefs

-3- meditate

Take these steps everyday for a month, then keep close watch over the events that begin to show up in your life.

Opportunities, information, direction, ideas, open doors will appear.

They will be the sign posts revealing the steps to the financial success you are waiting for. They will show you what to do next to change your financial life.

Because financial freedom is your birthright, it is not only possible; it is demanding you to let it come to you.

My greatest challenge was to stop taking money, more precisely, the lack thereof, so seriously.

What is your mindset about the money you want?

Is it that this is the most serious aspect of your life?

Is it that you'll never be able to get the money you need?

Is it that money problems rule?

Lighten up. Deliberately put a smile on your face and a light in your eye when you think about your money, no matter how non-existent your bank account is.

Sit in meditation with a smile on your face and a light in your eye and visualize (see chapter eight) every detail of your life with all the money you want in it.

Live in that world through your mind.

Remember that "mind is the creator of everything…if you cling to a certain thought…it finally assumes a tangible outward form…you become the controller of your destiny." Paramahansa Yogananda

Remember that "our only limitations are those we set up in our own minds". (Napolean Hill. <u>Think and Grow Rich</u>).

Be easy about money. Your wealth already exists, you are not separate from it.

It is on its way to you, just expect it, just allow it in.

Allow it first into your inner world, your mind, and then it will manifest in your outer world, your pocket.

RESOURCES

Creating Affluence. Deepak Chopra, Amber-Allen publishing, San Rafael, Calif. 1998.

Quantum Theology: Spiritual Implications of the New Physics. Diarmuid O'Murchu, Crossroads publishing, NY. 1998.

The Hidden Heart of the Cosmos. Brian Swimme, Orbis Books, Maryknoll, NY. 1996.

The Universe is a Green Dragon. Brian Swimme, Bear &Co., Santa Fe, New Mexico. 1984.

The Wealthy Barber. David Chilton, Prima Publishing, USA, 1996.

The Power of Now. Eckhart Tolle, Namaste Publishing, Vancouver, BC. 1997.

The Power of the Subconscious Mind. Joseph Murphy; Prentice Hall original edition, 1963. Bantam revised, 2001. USA and Canada.

Think and Grow Rich
The Science of Getting Rich
A Happy Pocket Full of Money
Wealth Consciousness
Spiritual Marketing

These five books are available as part of an e-book package called **Wealth Beyond Reason** at my website: www.diannepeck.com/ways to wealth.html

I'm Rich Beyond My Wildest Dreams I am, I am I am. Tom Pauley and Penelope Pauley.

Available as an ebook at www.richdreams.com and in paperback at www.amazon.com

Chapter Eight
Oh But You Can

Decide now to make your life grander, greater, richer and nobler than ever before.
Joseph Murphy

Oh but you can create the life you want. You can take that quantum leap into your best life. You are powerful and capable and you are the source of all that you need to make your heart's desires come true.

Everyone of us can stop feeling tossed around by the circumstances of our lives, and we can start operating from the driver's seat, even "at our age".

This is how to do that.

What do you want?

The very first thing to do is to decide what the precise desires of your heart are. What do you want to have show up in your life? What are your dreams? Do you still have any? Or has the "I'm getting too old for dreams" philosophy moved in when you weren't looking?

If so, go inside and recover your dreams. Your wishes and wants.

They are still there, they only wait to be brought out into the light and to live. They only wait to manifest themselves in your precious life. They only wait to take shape in your hands, to be felt and seen and smelled and tasted and heard.

Our dreams are reality and we are the keys to their incarnation, to giving them flesh.

At Our Age

That is such a huge point, we are the key to turning our dreams into reality.

We are the key; more precisely, our mind is the key.

It's all in how we use our mind, all in the thoughts we think.

You are the architect of your world, of your future, of your tomorrow.

No one has to say to you, "may the force be with you", because it is. It is more than with you, it is you.

Your money dreams, your relationship dreams, your career dreams, your retirement dreams, all wait for you to manifest them. So take step number one and get clear on what your dreams are.

The second thing you do is feel the passion for your dreams, feel it in your spirit.

A thought with feeling in it is an unstoppable force. It is the force that is required to get the job done. Think your dream and feel your dream as if it is already here and it is yours.

You may think your passion for your dreams has become faint-sounding, too long silent, a mere whisper, but it is still virile and fertile and will pulse again as soon as you put your attention on it.

Attention

Let's talk about attention.

In order to become the creator of our lives it is vital to be aware of what gets our attention. At our age it is not only bank machines that are automated, our thinking can be, too.

The majority of our thoughts can be comprised of assumptions, assumptions that our usefulness has waned, that opportunity no longer has any doors with our name on them, that nothing can change, that the movers and shakers are all under forty, that there are no more options.

Don't settle for unexamined assumptions.

They are not truth, but they can have that kind of power over us because they come from the "Land of They" (*Your Heart's Desire* by Sonia Choquette).

The Land of They controls our lives if we do not examine what "They" say, if we do not become the Liege of our own land.

You are the Liege of your mid-life years, and of all your years. You set the level of expectation. You make the rules about what can and cannot be done. You are the map-maker, charting your own course, and you are the helmsman, guiding yourself to your destination.

And just in case you are wondering just what attention has to do with creating your dreams, attention has everything to do with it because, the results we get come from the thoughts we think, so it follows that we need to become aware of which thoughts we are giving our attention to.

For example, a rampant fear in the Land of They is the fear of retirement.

The perception is that if I retire I will have nothing to do, that my potential flees, that new ideas are no longer in the realm of possibility, that I will no longer have an identity.

But this is the point about retirement: it is the top step on the success ladder, not the first step back to the bottom.

It is the showroom to the world of all those years of product testing and manufacturing, and that superb product is you. Here you are, rich with life-experience, compassionate, emotionally mature, skilled in the nuances of human interaction, and ready to play. Congratulations.

If retirement is one of your issues, the first question to ask yourself is, "What is my retirement dream?"

Answer that, and then examine your thoughts. Are they exciting, verdant, hopeful thoughts that support your dream? They are the only kind of thoughts that will carry your dream across the ether and into your life. Put your attention on them.

Of course, there is also the point that the current practice in the North American marketplace of mandatory retirement at age sixty-five may need an overhaul.

When senior employees (like us) are terminated, so is the high level of skill and performance we have garnered, along with our wisdom and insight for planning, our expertise in managing personnel, and our capacity as mentors.

Many sixty-five-ers are a rich resource, and their dream is to continue in their current employment.

And of course there is a part of us that never qualifies for retirement.

Joseph Murphy, in *The Power of the Subconscious Mind,* rightfully admonishes us not to retire our mind. He writes,

"Be sure your mind never retires. Your mind must be like a parachute, it's of no use at all unless it opens up".

Paying attention to what our thoughts are doing means we are keeping our parachute open.

Here is the story one woman tells about the difference it made to her life when she became deliberate about where she was putting her attention.

"A longtime relationship that had been both a coveted friendship and a love affair had ended. The ending had been at best obscure, and had left me feeling incomplete. Many weeks, then many months had passed but every time

I wanted to take steps for better closure, I was overcome with the old barrage of symptoms that always assailed me whenever a hint of stress showed up in my life: loss of appetite, loss of sleep, etc. I always responded to these symptoms by assuming they were an indication that I should abandon the planned activity, for the good of my health. Best not to "put myself through that", I would say. But that decision only lengthened the list of "I can't's" in my life, and did nothing for the restlessness in my spirit.

Then one day I decided to apply the attention theory to this issue. What if I focus on the outcome I want, instead of on the stress symptoms? What if I agree to follow the leading of my spirit which is to ignore the knots in my stomach, to let the panic rage on, and to take steps to fulfill this particular desire of my heart?

A few weeks pass and then one beautiful August afternoon, a Sunday, I know what I want to do.

I drive the two and a half hours to the place in the

country, stomach knots in tow, where we had spent some of our happiest hours. I walk the fields and sit by the generations-old brook. I muse about the remnants of the homemade fence, one of the few remaining pieces of evidence of the thriving farm these fields had once been.

Was the purpose of the fence to keep cows, ready to give birth, from seeking the isolation of the thicker woods beyond? Or was it simply just a property demarcation?

The sun embraces me with its warmth and the blue sky bends low to greet me. One bird tarries with me and sings the while. The awe I had always held for these early farm settlers fills me now and I once again feel their spirits.

I linger long, as the beauty surrounding me reunites me with all the beauty that had been part of the relationship. It was in that beauty that I had once found a home and for these brief moments I find it again.

Although I will probably never come back to this setting, I know now that the gift it had been will always be alive in my spirit.

At Our Age

September, and another Sunday.

What? Drive to the town where he lives? Are you sure? Acknowledging the need for further closure, I decided I was sure, took my stomach knots and went.

My destination only an hour away this time, I drive past the house where he lives and the building where he works.

I park at the waterfront, among the goings and comings of the tourists, and just let myself be, just allow myself to feel what I am feeling. This is as much geographical proximity as I am ready for, and I am handling it well.

Gradually I join in the late afternoon calm as it settles over the landscape. I watch a solitary kayaker glide over the serene waters of the bay, and feel my heart increase its peace and its sense of completion.

October now, another month, another unexpected development. Back in his town with a mutual friend, this time I am ready for a personal encounter.

We are warmly welcomed. I am happy to find he

looks well…I had heard he had been ill. The three-way conversation is natural and comfortable.

I am aware of the grace that is softly falling on the moment, and of the fusing of the holes of sadness in my soul. I remember the line from somewhere that says even a broken bottle holds the traces of perfume. I make a decision to remember the perfume and not the shattered bottle."

The teller of this story does not know at this time what lies ahead for the relationship in question, but she knows she walked tall and elegant to this moment.

The cost to her of this re-connection was sleepless nights, loss of appetite, and fatigue.

The gain was peace for her memories and the final seal on the past. The gain was her readiness now to run freely into the many new beginnings that had been patiently beckoning to her from the other compartments of her life.

The point is, the more we practice deliberate attention, the more we choose what gets our attention, the more we will have our heart's desires.

It will become as natural a way to proceed through life as falling off a log, as the saying goes. And when the life we want is in place, the causes of our fear and anxiety no longer exist, and neither do there accompanying symptoms.

Intention

To return to the task at hand, which was naming the steps to take to create the life you want, the third step is to deliberately intend it.

Once you have focused your attention on what you want, then make it your intention.

For example, you have absolutely no doubt that what you most need is to make a major life change by retiring from your job. You are ready to put your attention squarely there. You are ready to focus on what retirement will mean for your life and not on how tough the transition will be.

You can transition the hard way or the easy way. The easy way is to latch on to your intention like a leech on a swimmer's leg. Here are a few ways to do that:

#1. Repeat present-tense affirmations.

For example, "I am retired and loving it". "I am transitioning with ease." "I love the freedom I have to choose what I want to do and where I want to go". "I am excited about the new life I am creating." I love the thrill of uncovering my untapped potential", etc.

Whatever retirement means to you, speak it, but in the present as if it was happening this moment. Keep your affirmations brief and repeat them many times a day.

Your conscious mind will probably object. It will

insist that this little practice is silly and not real.

But you are in charge of your mind. You know that your thoughts create your reality and you know which reality is best for you. It is just a matter of staying with it until your conscious mind catches on and comes into agreement.

This is a new way of using your mind, you are laying down new track, you have begun working your mind to harness its immense power, power that science has yet to fully measure.

To handle the objections that lurch to the forefront, simply tell your mind that it doesn't have to believe the affirmations, because it doesn't. Just keep repeating them, and, as with any repeated thought, they become beliefs.

And then your mind will stop putting up its what ifs and buts. It will stop balking and will align itself with your intention and then you are home free. That is when things begin to happen.

#2. Visualize your perfect retirement.

What are your new goals? Who are you with? Where do you go? What are you wearing? What are you smelling? What are you hearing? What do you talk about? Give at least five minutes a day to this exercise.

#3. Get the feeling going.

How do you feel? What does it feel like to be living your dream? How does freedom feel? How does adventure feel? How does travel feel? How does stress-free living feel? How do new horizons feel? Feel and walk and talk and think and be as if your dream is here now.

#4. Let go of the outcome.

Don't tell yourself that letting go is impossible or too hard to do. Tell yourself that letting go of the outcome is something you may never have done but something that will be exciting to try.

This is how easy it is. It is as easy as putting a roast in the oven and trusting the oven to take it from there; as easy as stepping on the gas pedal and trusting the engine to take over its job.

Of course you have already turned on the oven and put gas in the tank. That's what steps one, two and three are about. They lay the groundwork because the car or oven doesn't operate on magic; you have to set up the conditions necessary for them to perform. That's your role, then you let them do theirs.

And so to get your dream life going, after you put your attention on the outcome you want and after you visualize it and feel it, then you leave it alone.

You forget about it for awhile and just go back to your day and the tasks at hand. You let manifestation take place on its own terms, terms you can be confident will be perfect in timing and circumstance.

#5. Receive your dream.

Are you really ready for your dream to arrive? It is already here and waiting for you. Open yourself to it. Let it in.

Follow these steps every day and watch yourself glide gently and perfectly into your new existence.

Closing thoughts

Well, that about wraps things up. Take the action steps that are in this book and you will make today and the rest of your life your dynamite years. Your dream relationship, your dream bank account, your dream contribution to the world, your dream retirement, your dream job, are completely possible and depend only on you for their actualization.

At Our Age

You have an incredible power within, the power of your own mind. Build the life you want with it. Your potential has no limits and it all begins with your thoughts. To get different results than you have always gotten, start thinking in a different way. Put the negative experiences of your past behind you and create your future from the place of the person you are now. The abundance of creation awaits you.

Earlier this month I was filled with the anticipation of viewing a lunar eclipse which was to happen at approximately 9:15 pm for us in Atlantic Canada.

At 9:00 pm I scurried out of the grocery store and into an early winter squall, winds blasting and skies invisible. Disappointed but determined, I drove to the walking track, where the full moon is breathtakingly beautiful when the sky isn't churned up with storm clouds and whirling snow.

I sat in my car for about ten minutes, staring at the

opaque windshield, envisioning what was happening above and beyond the blizzard, and was just about ready to abandon my stakeout when I heard another car drive up.

Car doors opened and shut and voices exclaimed, "There it is, look!" I fairly leaped out of my blind.

From behind, wind and snow whipped at us and filled a menacing sky. But in front we gaped in disbelief at the view.

There, clouds had parted, stars shone, and a dark red, eclipsed moon silently hung.

And that is how possible it is for the inevitability of our lives, like the emulsified sky, to break open and reveal the wonders our lives seek and our hearts desire.

RESOURCES

Retirement and Career Coaching:

If your are transitioning into retirement now or want to plan for it now, contact Joanne Waldman, Director of Training for Retirement Options.

Joanne is especially qualified as a Retirement coach. Her coaching process includes using the Retirement Success Profile (RSP) assessment tool, which addresses the fifteen factors necessary for successful retirement.

Get coached by phone from the comfort of your own home or office.

Contact Information:

Phone: 314-469-3288

Email: joanne@newperspectivecoaching.com

Website: www.newperspectivecoaching.com

<u>Your Heart's Desire: Instructions For Creating the Life You Really Want.</u> Sonia Choquette, Three Rivers Press, New York. 1997.

Appendix A
Taking Action

Here is a list of the Action Steps that are given in this book:

Chapter Two: Page
The OK List   25
The Success Lifeline   32
Getting Connected   34
Self-Care Tips   38

Chapter Three:
Mind Your Mind   48
Breathing Technique   60
Meditation - morning pages   56

Chapter Four:
Live in the Moment   70
Gratitude Note Book   83

Chapter Five:

Pleasure List	94
Overcome Loneliness	97
Proceed As If	101
Make Plans (Be in Love)	102

Chapter Eight:

Pay Attention to Your Desire	164
Intend Your Desire (five steps)	173

More Action Steps

The Creation Box

The creation box is a fun way to get focused on what you want. Get a box, a shoebox is fine, and decorate it to give it special significance, or purchase a decorated one in the stationary department.

Now clip pictures of your wants and dreams, or write them on notes, or doodle or draw them. Represent them in some way and put them in the box.

Your requests can be as mundane as a nice comfortable but inexpensive brand of pen (which I needed for my writing and which I immediately located after months of trying many not-comfortable ones), or as grandiose as winning the lotto.

In doing this you are focusing and visualizing and paying attention in a powerful way to what you want to manifest.

And results are phenomenal. You will be thrilled at how quickly you will start taking the notes back out of the box because their contents have already shown up.

And of course you just keep adding more images as the need arises.

Play in your Creation Box often.

<u>Creation Board</u>

You can follow the same principles of the Creation Box only post your pictures and drawings and notes on a Creation Board, a bulletin board which you can see daily and which acts as a reminder of your positive expectations.

Positive Aspect Notebook

Get a small fun notebook and each evening write five things you appreciate about the day and what transpired in it.

In so doing you are fostering Albert Sweitzer's understanding of the power of an attitude of gratitude. He wrote, "You must learn to understand the secret of gratitude. It is more than just so-called virtue. It is revealed as a mysterious law of existence".

Ways to "Proceed as if"

If you are working at having your perfect lover show up in your life, clean your apartment/house now, improve it now, learn to cook now, or buy those romantic candles or a piece of lingerie now.

If you are working at getting a large amount of money, give some away, in an amount you can afford.

I know of some who do it this way. They pick a name and address at random from the telephone directory, then address an envelope and put money in it. Included is an anonymous note explaining how they selected the receiver's name, and that they are doing this because they believe that by creating abundance for others they draw it to themselves.

How's that for an act of wild abandon.

Appendix B
The Power of Allowing

This is a talk I gave at the Annual Celebration of Remembrance that has been held for the last fourteen years by our local Hospice/Palliative Care organization, for those whose family member died during the past year.

It is purposely held in early December with the specific goal of easing the pain of transition, which is especially harsh during the holiday season.

I include it here because it outlines the way out of grief, one of life's most demanding transitions.

The Power of Allowing

To begin our reflection I would like to invite you, for the next few minutes, to focus on relaxing.

Let your shoulders drop and let the weight of your body sink into your chair.

Breathe in and out slowly a few times.

Do not strain to listen. Just allow yourself to be present to the words.

Then if there is a word here for your heart, it will just stick to it all on its own.

Major life transitions come to us in many forms.

Life can jump up and change on us sometimes without much notice. We can feel that life has betrayed us.

Two years ago I faced major changes in my life, that put me in a position of living on my own for the first time, and of needing employment.

So I began to study for a career as a Life Coach.

I have named my business, <u>Oh But You Can Coaching</u>.

At Our Age

I chose that name because they were the words I most needed to hear.

Because I was in danger of letting "I can't do this" take over my life.

And because I was learning that I didn't have to let that happen.

If you have lost someone you love and who loved you, you're in a major life transition.

Maybe thoughts such as, "I can't do this".

"I don't want to do this."

"I don't want to make it" are at times what you are thinking and feeling.

And maybe when those thoughts come, you try to bury them or you feel alarmed by them, or in one way or another you censor them.

There is a much gentler way to make it through transition.

Here it is.

Our feelings originate with a thought. That's how we are constructed.

When you become aware of the thought that has dug into your mind with jaws of steel, do this one thing.

Say to the panic, or the anger, or the guilt, or the desperation, or the uncertainty or the fear that you are thinking and feeling,

Say, "Panic, it is alright that you are here".

That may not be the answer you were expecting.

"Too simple", you may be thinking.

It is simple, and it is powerful.

We call it allowing. You allow whatever you are thinking to be what it is, and to be with you.

This is a way to be extremely loving and gentle toward yourself, by allowing your thoughts and the feelings that come with them to be with you.

If you belong to the human race, you have the

whole possible range of human thoughts at your fingertips, like it or not.

In her book, *The Places That Scare You,* author Pema Chodron tells us to be like the mother bird protecting and feeding her "naked, squawking homely babies".

The thing is this.

Our troubling thoughts are like new chicks demanding to be attended to.

And we are the mother bird gathering them in, in all their noise and homeliness, with unconditional love. With love and gentleness.

I promise you that when we do that, two things happen.

The first thing is, the thoughts and feelings that have commandeered our life begin to settle down. Like chicks, they begin to grow up.

This is because we have given them what they had been seeking, a rightful place with us.

The second thing that happens is this.

Instead of being a massive drain on our energy, they become transformed into new energy for us.

An energy that surprises us.

An energy we thought we had lost forever.
As we become easier with this allowing process, the pain changes.

It becomes a new spirit in our day.

This is a fragile new spirit at first, and delicate.

You may be familiar with this endearing line from the Talmud, the sacred writings of Judaism.

At Our Age

"Every blade of grass has its angel bending over it and whispering, 'Grow. Grow'."

Every blade of grass, plain, simple, who-even-notices blade of grass has its own angel.

That's a lot of angels.

I don't know if every blade of grass has its angel.

I think the point is that whether or not we believe in angels, what we are doing when we allow our thoughts, whatever they are, to be with us, when we give them a place with us, when we pour gentleness over ourselves in this way, what we are doing is becoming our own angel, we are bending over our own broken-ness.

We are whispering to that small and frail blade of new life that is beginning in us, and what we are saying is:

"Yes, you can make it. You are doing so well. I am so proud of you."

Appendix C
Life Coaching

Coaching in itself is not a new concept.

We are very much at home with the idea of drama, voice, music, athletic or corporate coaching.

In the corporate world today, survey stats show that 60% of companies support management by some form of coaching, and 20% will be ready to jump on board within a year.

Specialization in the coaching profession is no longer confined to the executive or the athletic world and now includes the personal, career, and relationship areas of our lives.

Personal (Life) Coaching is the second fastest growing industry in the US, burgeoning in Australia, progressing at a good clip in Europe, and quietly infiltrating Canada.

There are an estimated 40,000 coaches worldwide and the profession is increasing at 20% per year.

History of Coaching

Explanations for the explosion are found in its history.

The roots of Life Coaching were formed when, according to Dr. Patrick Williams and Deborah Davis in their book, "Therapist as Life Coach", psychiatry's traditional perspective of seeing the client as being sick and the therapist as the fixer of the client's problems, began to give way to seeing the therapist as being the catalyst to help the client find the solutions within himself or herself.

"Psychological theorists in the early part of the 20th century set the framework for life coaching's 'whole and healthy person' view. The shift from seeing clients as ill or pathological toward viewing them as 'well and whole' and seeking a richer life is paramount to understanding the evolution of life coaching"(Williams p.11).

So what is the difference between coaching and therapy or consulting?

The three disciplines are related because they share common origins, but each has a distinct purpose.

The purpose of therapy is to make us functional.
The purpose of consulting is to give us solutions.
The purpose of coaching is to take us from an already-functional place, to one where we uncover our own strengths and our own solutions.

Therapy and counseling deal with the past in order to create a healthy present.

Coaching deals with the future in order to create the life we desire.

International Coaching Federation

The International Coaching Federation (ICF) defines coaching as a relationship that helps people produce extraordinary results in their lives, careers, businesses, or organizations.

ICF is the international body that sets the ethical standards for the coaching profession, and grants the highest levels of Certification.

Today there are close to fifty coach training schools worldwide.

What Coaching Is

Coaching is a dialogue between you and your coach for the purpose of getting you to where you have decided you want to be in your life.

And if you aren't clear yet on where it is you need to be but know that it is no longer where you are, coaching can solve that problem too.

Coaching is a partnership based on mutual agreements which give structure and support to your life.

Coaching is a process with a unique power to tap into all your strengths and into all the answers you need.

The coaching process finds those strengths and answers where they already are, inside your own mind and your own knowing.

Coaching is unique because it operates from the premise that your own wisdom is more than you need and that you already have it.

Getting a Life Coach belongs in your "best thing I ever did for myself" file.

What Coaching Is Not

Coaching is not counseling, consulting, or therapy. The focus of these disciplines is past events that still impact our lives now.

The focus of coaching is the present in order to define, articulate and organize it so it can take us to the future.

The purpose of coaching is to create the life you want.

Coaching is future-based. A coach stays with you after the goals are written down. A coach stays until S-Day, the day you celebrate Success.

At Our Age

Who Needs A Coach?

You need a Life Coach if you want to:

- establish direction in any area of your life
- set and reach exciting goals
- increase your capacity for happiness
- get organized and clutter free
- practice excellent personal management
- transition to a new career
- change your lifestyle or your self-image
- start a new relationship or recreate an old one
- fulfill personal and business commitments
- re-stoke your life-passion or uncover a new one
- be free from limiting beliefs, self-defeating patterns, unfulfilling work

About Me

I am a coach who believes in the individual greatness of each person.

I believe in Plato's words, "Take charge of your thoughts. You can do what you will with them".

I believe in our capacity to take charge of our thoughts to create the life we want.

I believe any circumstance can be altered to the good.

I believe we can't get it wrong.

I believe coaching is the most fulfilling career I could be in.

Other careers I have loved are teaching, both youth and adults; co-ordinating and leading life-skills seminars; raising a family.

My avocation is writing.

My goal as a Life Coach is to be:
- a map-maker, navigating you from where

you are to where you need to go
- a companion to walk you through transitions, challenges, and goals
- a holder of your potential, your passion, and your dream

Coaching Credentials

- I am trained by the International Coaching Academy (ICA), a state-of-the-art learning facility staffed by industry leaders.
- I am currently earning International Certification.
- I am a member of Coachville, the leading governing body for the professional coaching industry.

Find Out More:

Dianne Peck

Oh But You Can Coaching

www.diannepeck.com

coach@diannepeck.com

ph/fax: 902-562-7982

About the Author

Life Coach and author Dianne Peck understands firsthand the challenges mid-life can bring. Dianne re-made her life two years ago.

Her story was featured on the national television program "2nd Chance: Making it Work".

Making it work is what she is doing, and what she wants to show you how to do. You are the perfect age to create your life like a newly-minted dime. Dianne named her coaching business *Oh But You Can Coaching* because "those were the words I most needed to hear. I was in danger of letting 'I can't' take over my life".

Printed in the United States
24719LVS00006B/1-69